NATURALLY SEXY & HEALTHY

DOCTOR LYNN WYLNN

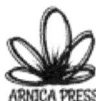

ARNICA PRESS

The material contained in this book has been written for informational purposes and is not intended as a substitute for medical advice, nor is it intended to diagnose, treat, cure, or prevent disease. If you have a medical issue or illness, consult a qualified physician.

Published by ARNICA PRESS

www.ArnicaPress.com

ARNICA PRESS

Copyright © 2010, 2022 Doctor Lynn Wylnn

www.DoctorLynn.com

Printed in the United States of America.

ISBN: 978-1-955354-17-2

The SOUL WALKING *Series*

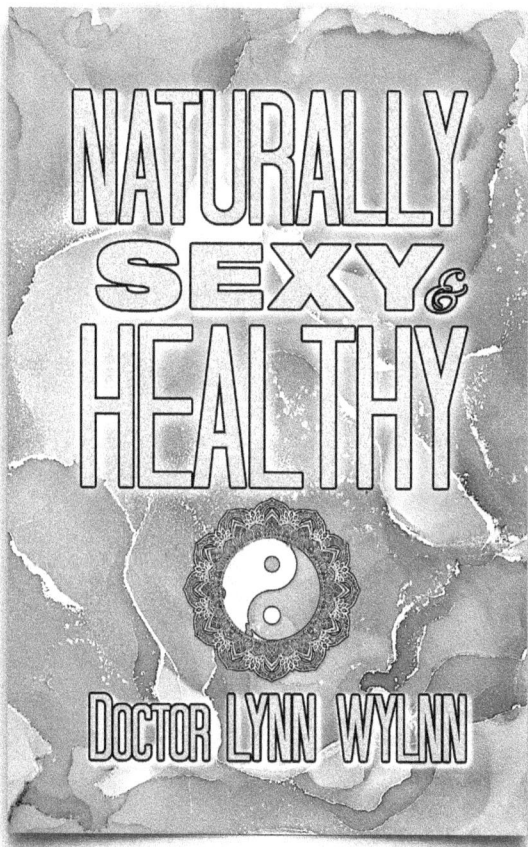

NATURALLY SEXY & HEALTHY

Doctor LYNN WYLNN

BOOK FOUR

BY DOCTOR LYNN WYLNN

THE SOUL WALKING SERIES:

HOW TO MASTER KARMA

HOW TO PROSPER WITH A PURPOSE

HOW TO MASTER VITALITY

HOW TO MASTER BURNOUT

NATURALLY SEXY AND HEALTHY

RECIPES FOR HEALTH, SEX, HAPPINESS AND LOVE

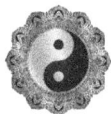

*Thank you to my husband Dan,
for supporting and encouraging me to write this book.
A special thanks to all my students and friends
who have been the source of my inspiration and a special thank you
to Arnica Press for all the guidance, suggestions and encouragement.*

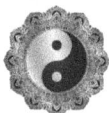

TABLE OF CONTENTS

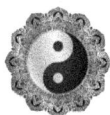

PREFACE

I'm a female, a daughter, a woman, a mother, a grandmother, a wife, and a cancer survivor. This book is the result of all the sexual aspects of my life. For, you see, my sexuality is at the heart of each of the many passages throughout my life.

In 2008, I underwent a radical hysterectomy because of cancer. It was a radical change both to my body and my mind. Although cancer hits everyone with such a jolt, it had a deeper and pervasive fear for me. My mother had been diagnosed with cancer when she was quite young and had undergone a radical hysterectomy. Her sense of womanhood had been invaded at a young age. I had grown up with this disease. In her day, little was known about hormones, diet, and exercise, and how these simple healthy lifestyle changes could affect both moods and energy. Relationships were not discussed and very little counseling was available. My mother was pretty much left alone with her emptiness.

Because of the hysterectomy she never menstruated beyond the age of twenty-five. We never shared this part of being a woman. I was told that she was not interested in sex and had lost all desire and drive. I later learned this was not true. There is more to drive and desire than retaining your sexual organs.

My mother did try to suppress my sexuality. I suppose she was somewhat jealous of my youthful bloom and her fading glow. I think all mothers must feel this way. She also feared that I would get pregnant. I was raised in New England in a very Victorian-minded family where issues of sex and emotions were not to be discussed. I, on the other hand, was very adventuresome and outspoken. I'm a baby boomer and an ex-hippie from the generation of free love.

My greatest fear as I was growing up was that I would get cancer and have my womanhood snatched from me. So when I was diagnosed with cancer three years into a new marriage, I went into a panic. Not only did I have cancer throughout my entire pelvic region, but I would suddenly be thrown into menopause and rendered sexless (or so I thought). Behind the fear of cancer lay a deeper fear. I would lose my sexuality and become the cold, empty woman I had imagined my mother to be.

I escaped the fate of my mother until the age of fifty-five when cancer came calling. Menopause, which I had planned to go through naturally, was suddenly being thrust upon me. There was no time to think or to plan. Like most women of my generation, I believed that menopause was the end of sex. Women, it was believed, simply lost the desire, shriveled up, and got old. I have since learned that oftentimes it is the man who loses the ability and the desire, leaving the woman to ponder her fate. Why do you think Viagra sales have soared? Sexual desire and sexual interest does not stop with menopause or age. It is something that we retain our entire lives. Our sexuality and our desire to love and make love go with us to the end.

I buried my deepest fears, never to speak of them, until now. For one year before my diagnosis I was sick. I was bleeding without knowing why, losing weight, achy and tired. However, every Pap smear and biopsy came back clean. Cancer is like that. It can escape diagnosis and disguise itself as something else. The doctors called it menopause and stress.

I was under a lot of stress. I was two years into a new marriage. I had waited 25 years to get remarried. Over that 25 years, I had struggled from a place of having nothing to educating myself, raising and educating my children, and establishing a very self-sufficent life. Then I met my husband. We believed we were meant for each other and, against my better judgment, we got married. He was newly divorced for the third time. We fought like

NATURALLY SEXY & HEALTHY ~ Doctor Lynn Wylnn

most newly married couples as we struggled to adjust. However, we had the extra stress of exes and children. My marriage was unstable and falling apart. I was tired and stressed. We were on the verge of a divorce. And then I was diagnosed with cancer. My husband held me and told me he would stand by me. I wondered if it was out of a sense of obligation, pity, or guilt. He was now stuck with a wife diagnosed with cancer and a very shaky marriage. I felt so bad for him. What would be left for him? I was either going to die or be rendered a sexless, middle-aged woman. I cried alone in the early morning hours when no one could hear me.

I had to tell my children and my family. Those were the hardest calls to make. I broke down crying. I could not be strong, even though I knew for my children I had to appear hopeful. The cancer was in my cervix and uterus. There were cysts on my ovaries. No one was sure if those were cancerous or not. I was covered with endometriosis. No one was sure if it had moved into my lymph nodes. Everything must go, including about 22 lymph nodes. They call it a radical hysterectomy.

I had to tell my students. I choked up as I told class after class that I had cancer and had to leave for six to eight weeks, but I insisted I would be back to teach. There was horror and fear on their faces. When you know someone who gets diagnosed with cancer, it sends a chill up your spine. If it can happen to them, it can happen to you. People back away because they don't know what to say. They are afraid of the disease and afraid of hurting you. So they avoid eye contact and conversations. You feel it. It's like they think if they get near you they'll catch it, too. It's very lonely. The surgery was scheduled for two weeks from the diagnosis. I continued to teach up until the day before the surgery. I remember teaching my yoga class and wondering if I would ever be able to teach again. I cried silent tears as my students rested in Savasana. In my cycle class I played a song by Rhianna, *Don't Stop the Music*. I cried. I did not want the music to stop. I played another song by Jem, *Keep on Walking*. God, give me the strength to keep on walking.

The day after the surgery all I could do was get out of bed with the help of a nurse and sit in a chair for five minutes. The pain was beyond anything I had ever experienced. I could not walk, let alone dance, do yoga, or cycle. I could not think about my sexuality, my children, and my husband or anything but my recovery. It would be long and arduous. And I was not out of the woods. Remission was two long years away.

I am a petite and rather thin woman. I lost five pounds the year before diagnosis, which is a lot of weight on my small frame. I weighed 95 pounds. I lost 10 pounds after the surgery. After the surgery, between the pain and the drugs, I couldn't eat. The day I came home from the hospital, I stood naked in front of the mirror. My body was wasted and emaciated except for a swollen and protruding abdomen, marked with a scar from hipbone to hipbone. I stood in front of the mirror and cried. Thanks to medical marijuana, I was able to get off the narcotics and begin eating. I gained back five of the 10 pounds I lost.

Right after the surgery, I lay in bed unable to move. For the first time in my life, I knew what it felt like to not be able to get out of bed. I could not move, and I could not walk for two days. Then I got out of bed, took about five steps, and collapsed in pain. Determined to get back on my feet, each day I would get out of bed and, in agony, drag my body, attached to an IV and catheter, down the hospital corridor and back to my bed. I was going to regain my strength.

At home, I got dressed every day with a lot of effort. I dragged myself around the house. Starting at two weeks, I went for a short walk. I walked a block to the bus stop and collapsed on the bench. I cried in fear that I could not make it back home. Just a month before I taught two classes a day, and now I couldn't walk a block. But each day I walked a little more. Slowly, I regained my strength. At eight weeks, I returned to teaching my classes. I remember the fear I felt. I was so afraid that I would not be able to teach class. All my wonderful students were so supportive and appreciative. I did not teach a full class, but slowly, and with a lot of determination, worked my way back into a strong and happy soul. Over the first year I struggled to regain my strength. After teaching a class, I would go home and need to rest. But I persisted and never once let anyone see me cry or feel sorry for myself. I did all of that alone.

I am now two years into my recovery. So far, no signs of cancer. I am strong, happy, having fun and my marriage is better than ever. My life is good, and I appreciate every moment. I did not turn into a cold and sexless woman. Quite the contrary. That's why I wrote this book. Because sex *does* matter. It is the essence of life.

The difference between those who enjoy their sexuality and those who don't is a matter of health and outlook. It is the driving force behind all of life. Sex sells. Sex gets our attention. We never stop the desire, even if the ability and opportunity has passed us by.

Anyone who has been diagnosed with cancer and gone through the arduous struggle of recovery knows the fear that lingers on through the first year into recovery. Every ache, every pain, every doctor's visit is cause for alarm. The fear lingers beneath the tough veneer that you put on for others and for yourself. The exhaustion and fear remind you daily that at any moment the cancer can return and your life can go upside down.

As a cancer survivor, I have learned the importance of embracing life. It is only when life is threatened that we truly appreciate the grand design of things. My sexuality is stronger than it was before my cancer. That is because my outlook is positive, fun-loving and embracing. I appreciate my energy and my ability to move and dance. I laugh as often and as loud as I can. I appreciate many things; most of all the opportunity to love and be loved.

Sexuality is more than just the physical act. It's a perception, an outlook, the way you carry yourself and the way you interact. Sexuality is more than your sexual organs. It's an attitude and it all begins in the mind. Does sex matter? You bet it does! Is health important? Absolutely! Combine a healthy body-mind with a sexy attitude and you have charisma, success, and the foundation of a happy and successful life.

My wish for you is that somewhere in this book you find that spark of magic that keeps the fires burning and the love for life blooming.

Doctor Lynn

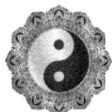

INTRODUCTION

I am not an authority on the subject of sex and pleasure but simply an observer, curious about what makes us tick. I am a naturopath who believes that sexual health is essential to a happy life.

Does sex matter? You bet it does! Everything in life involves some element of sex. Without sex, not only would life cease to exist, but passion would die, art would disappear, and just about everything that makes the world revolve would wither and fade.

When I was in my undergraduate study, I took an elective course called human sexuality. I was a young woman, divorced with two children, and thought I could breeze through the course. Little did I know that I was about to get an education that would make even an experienced person sit up and take notice. The class was held at night in a large auditorium. The room was full, with 100 students. The lights were low, and the stage was lit. Out onto the stage walked a rather frumpy middle-aged man. He was notably short, not very good-looking, but strong and bold in his presentation. The first thing he said was that there was only one thing for us to remember, "The very first thing you are is a sexual being. You are either male or female. Your sexuality defines you before you take form."

To me this was very profound. I had never thought about life, sex, or being in such fundamental terms. He went on to tell us that everything in life is driven by sex. Everything we do, create, and desire has somewhere in it an element of sex. Sex sells! Watch car commercials, laundry detergent commercials, look at magazine ads...everything is designed to make us look better, feel better, and be better; and thereby instills desire.

Sex has many faces, desires, fantasies, and orientations. It starts out as the simple infusion of egg and sperm and then mushrooms into a myriad of expressions.

Sex takes on many roles in our lives. It starts out with curiosity and then moves on to raging hormones, copulation, procreation, adventure, experience, eroticism, making love, and gratification. Of all the human drives, it is the most profound. Humans will give up food and water, shelter, money, health, and life for the momentary expression of sex. Look around you and you will see sex everywhere. The biggest-selling item on the Internet is sex! Why do you think Viagra sales soared? Because sex is fundamentally one of life's greatest pleasures and none of us want to lose it.

Sexual expression is about pleasure and delight. It is play, affection, touching, and desiring. It makes us feel alive, full of energy, and young. The excitement of sexual attraction lifts our spirits, makes life seem bright, and makes us feel on top of the world. Take away that spark and the world seems dull and cold. That is why we all constantly seek sensual desire. It does something chemically to our brains that is so powerful and feels so good that we seek it over and over again. Add love to the equation and we have the cocktail of ecstasy.

But sadly, many times people enter into relationships without thinking through the long-term compatibilities. They become so caught up in the sex and the excitement that they simply don't look at the basis of a loving and healthy relationship: namely compatibility, understanding, respect, caring, compassion, and appreciation. Many things will happen over time and the test of a relationship and its sexual health will depend upon forgiveness, understanding, and compassion.

Many people enter into relationships for reasons other than love: to end loneliness, fear of not finding someone else, fill a gap, money, social status, ego gratification, to end depression, for sex, to recover from a previous relationship, family pressure, or to end boredom. None of these will sustain a healthy sex life or bring love. Only commitment, maturity, sharing, and compatibility will renew the fires of desire as sex waxes and wanes throughout time.

As we age, the experience of sexual pleasure takes on a different meaning. We seek more than simple physical expression. Fucking leaves us empty, where lovemaking renews us and connects us on all levels: body, mind, and soul.

Because most people don't understand the nature of spiritual love, they become bound in the illusion of the physical world. Pleasures of the senses and of the flesh supersede a deeper spiritual experience. Pleasure is not "bad." It is part of the process of being human. Sadly, the momentary pleasures seem to leave us emptier and emptier. That is why the accumulation of material wealth has never brought eternal happiness.

Sex matters. It begins with a healthy body-mind that expands beyond the momentary pleasures of sex and enters into the depth of sexual lovemaking. It is here that the spiritual element of sex enters and it is said we achieve the ultimate in ecstasy. The Buddha reminded us that, when we are on the spiritual path, we cannot ignore our health. The path teaches us a reverence for the temple of the soul or the body-mind and, wanting to experience the greatest expression of your sensual and sexual self, you will seek that which enhances. It begins with an understanding of the nature of our sexuality and how to enrich it through a lifestyle where pleasure is associated with the ideals of a long and healthy life: radiance, happiness, wisdom, physical vitality, adaptability, sexual vigor and response, mental acuity, anti-aging, love-compassion, and a harmonious relationship with nature and other human beings.

May you find within these pages the majestic, the lore, and the secret of sexual matters, and everlasting pleasures.

Doctor Lynn

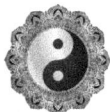

~ A successful life: to give and receive affection and love. ~

IT IS A LITTLE BIOCHEMISTRY
AND MORE...

Sex is about the most natural thing we do and, yet, we complicate it. We worry about performance, duration, satisfaction, and multiple orgasms. In all the pressure to have great sex, we forget about the natural aspect of our sexual nature. We are sexual beings designed with a hormonal system that requires a nutritionally sound body-mind to perform at maximum capacity. It is all so natural and, yet, we complicate it by searching for satisfaction through different positions, pornography, and multiple partners. With a better understanding of our sexual health, we can reach heights of ecstasy using the gifts nature has bestowed upon us.

So let us start by looking at the sexual being. We are born either male or female and, from there, we discover our sexual orientation. Whatever our leaning, it is the hormonal biochemistry that starts the engine of drive and desire. In addition to testosterone and estrogen there are other chemicals fueling the sexual fire. We are a complex structure of biology and chemistry fed by the nature of arriving in the world a living being.

Biochemistry is the chemistry of living things. Human beings function based upon the chemistry or makeup of their communication system. Hormones and peptides drive the basic instincts and desires of the body-mind. We now know that a mixture of hormones circulating in the body at any given time will determine (somewhat) how you respond to your lover or a new attraction, your emotional reaction, how sexy and turned-on you feel, your inclination to commit, and much more about the nature of our sensual and sexual dance. When you fall in love, touch, get excited, or feel desire, certain hormones are at work while other hormones take a back seat. The mixture of hormones at work determines how you feel, what you think, and how you act.

Although this may be a bit academic, it is important to understand the biochemistry of our sexuality in order to discover the natural ways to enhance our desires and drives. An understanding of this will show you how our hormones and peptides work to excite and unite. I'll try to keep it simple so this quick biochemistry lesson will be as sweet as bees to honey.

I hope this book will make you think about the nature of your sexual self and how simple things like diet and exercise can improve your sex life. First, we need to meet the arsenal of hormones and peptides that make up our sexual chemical soup. Each has a role to play; and some, when combined, can explain a multitude of thoughts, actions, drives, and desires.

So let's meet our friends and together see if we can begin to explore that nature of you, me, and these things called lust, love, and sex.

Meet our friends: DHEA, pheromones, oxytocin, PEA, estrogen, testosterone, serotonin, dopamine, progesterone, prolactin, and vasopressin. This mixture of hormones and peptides are what drives us and deters us from sexual and sensual pleasure. Each plays a role to bring about balance and order. However, when one is low and another is high, all kinds of things can happen. We can go from raging to bottoming out. They drive our desires, basic instincts, and emotional makeup. So let us get a quick lesson on the nature of our biochemistry. DHEA — there is more DHEA in your body (male or female) than any other hormone. DHEA is called the "mother of all hormones" because most of our other hormones are derived from it. It tells us when we can and cannot have sex. Animal studies indicate that DHEA is involved in sex drive, orgasm, and sex appeal.

DHEA is produced primarily by the adrenal glands. Both men and women have nearly equal amounts, except in the brain. The brain can make its own DHEA and, in fact, levels of DHEA are higher in the human brain than any other sex hormone. DHEA and testosterone share similar properties. They are both male hormones and androgens. It is important to note that DHEA is primarily produced in the brain and that women have more DHEA in the brain than men. It is believed this is in part due to the influence of testosterone, which outnumbers DHEA in men.

Women seem to derive the greatest benefits from DHEA. In the late 1950s, DHEA was identified as a sex hormone in females. A study at the Sloan- Kettering Cancer Research Institute on women whose ovaries had been

removed because of cancer revealed that their sex drives were still intact. If the ovaries were removed and estrogen was no longer being produced, what could account for the continued sex drive? The researchers concluded that the DHEA made by the adrenal glands, along with testosterone and other substances, were responsible. In addition, the women were no longer producing progesterone (the anti–sex-drive hormone), so more DHEA was available to ignite the fire. Cancer patients who had both the ovaries and the adrenal glands removed showed a significant drop in sex drive and desire. Only in female humans, as opposed to other mammals, can the ovaries be removed and the sex drive stays intact. The conclusion from this is that the shift from female hormones to male hormones (androgens/DHEA) occurs.

DHEA may also influence women more than men where sexual desire and body image intersect. DHEA affects your fat metabolism in a positive way. It helps you stay thin! It triggers a "futile fatty-acid cycle" that raises your metabolic thermostat, causing you to burn more energy. The less fat in your flesh, the more you produce DHEA; and the more fat, the lower your DHEA.

Some things in our daily life affect the level of DHEA. It increases with puberty, prolactin, bupropion (an antidepressant), exercise, meditation, smoking, digoxin, and sex. It decreases with alcohol, aging, chronic illness, obesity, anorexia nervosa, autoimmune disease, and certain medications.

Right now, the U.S. does not approve DHEA supplements. Therefore, it is best at this time to avoid naturally what decreases DHEA and include what naturally increases DHEA into your life. I would propose that certain things like cigarette smoking be avoided; but exercise, meditation, and sex along with losing weight and staying stress-free can go a long way to increasing DHEA.

Our next friend in the hormone soup is pheromones. Pheromones are derived from DHEA. Pheromones are sexual signals transmitted through the sense of smell from one individual to another. In the animal kingdom, pheromones dictate the mating dance. There is no conscious thought, only the primal instinct of scent. In humans, it is a subliminal effect. DHEA plays a major role in the subliminal effects of pheromones.

DHEA has a maternal role in that, with the sense of smell (pheromones) and the sense of touch, a baby bonds with its mother. Studies have indicated that women have a higher sense of smell and touch than men, which might be caused by the increased DHEA in the brain. The sense of smell is related to estrogen, and since women have more estrogen than men do, their sense of smell is more acute.

Pheromones affect men and women differently. Those that influence women do not influence men and vice versa. Instead of causing irresistible sex drive and desire in humans (as they do with animals), the pheromones appear to influence sensuality, well-being, and intimacy.

It is important to note that each of us has our own "smell print." Our scent is unique. When we move around, we leave a scent behind. This is because our skin is awash with unique molecules and when we slough off skin, we leave behind our unique smell. Police use the clothing from individuals and dogs to detect a person's scent.

We will discuss pheromones later on in the book when we explore the sense of smell and our sexuality.

Oxytocin is my favorite molecule. It influences our relationships through the sense of touch. It is the glue that binds us. When someone touches you, your oxytocin levels rise. Moreover, if that someone is someone you are attracted to or love, your levels will really rise! Oxytocin bonds and attaches us to those we love such as mates, friends, family, and babies. It is a big part of parenting behavior, causes contractions during birth and orgasms, reduces stress, and most importantly keeps us touching each other in tender and loving ways. Curiously, oxytocin also makes us forgetful and diminishes our reasoning capacity.

PEA, the molecule of love, is the nectar of romance. When you experience that falling-in-love state of being, PEA is probably at work. PEA, short for *phenylethylamine*, is a naturally occurring amphetamine substance that makes you feel as if you are walking on air, out of touch, and with your head in the clouds. It is found in chocolate, diet soft drinks, and in the bloodstream of lovers. It mimics diet pills, which might explain why some people lose their appetite when falling in love. And it spikes during orgasm!

Some people get so addicted to the high of PEA that they become love junkies, moving from one love to the next. Some people even think that lovesickness could be because of a drop in PEA levels in the bloodstream.

Estrogen is the sexy curvy kitten inside each of us. It is responsible for softness both in body and in mind. We get playful, alluring, and emotional on estrogen. Men are always attracted to the essence of estrogen. Maybe it is because estrogen develops the breast and endows a woman with the bodily aspects of sex appeal. The way a woman smells and her sense of smell is greatly influenced by estrogen. Remember pheromones? Women have more estrogen, so their sense of smell is stronger. With estrogen flowing, a woman opens her arms and begs for penetration. Estrogen directs her receptive sex drive and makes her surrender to the man perusing her driven by his testosterone.

Testosterone is what makes a man a man. It is the sexual, sensual, dark, and dangerous subtlety of a man. Testosterone is responsible for the aggressive sex drive. It is the fuel that gives us drive, determination, initiation, and domination. It also stimulates the production of dopamine, which is associated with the pleasure center.

Testosterone seems to have more of an effect on drive as opposed to frequency and potency.

Testosterone is also known for aggression, violence, and competitiveness. Most of these traits are associated with men because they happen to have more testosterone than women do. It is an aphrodisiac of sorts for both sexes as it promotes the drive for intercourse, orgasm, and procreation.

Testosterone is a double-edged sword; it drives us to lust, but also causes us to be aggressive, irritable, and overbearing and to be loners. It makes us want sex, but also to be alone and in control of sexual situations. It promotes masturbation and one-night stands. Testosterone is the basic drive with no emotional entanglements. It surges with conquest and acquisition of power, but once the conquest is made, it is on to the next! Men driven by testosterone will copulate without thought, whereas women, who have less testosterone and need more intimacy, are less willing to engage in one-night stands.

In addition, one further thing: testosterone spikes over a monthly period (just like women and estrogen). It can make a man angry and irritable.

Serotonin is a neurotransmitter, which means it acts to relay signals in your brain from one nerve ending to another. When serotonin levels are high, we are sensitive and peaceful, with sex drive diminishing. When levels are low, sex drive, as well as aggression and depression, spikes. In fact, when levels are low, we may become inhibited sexually, as well as violent and mean. Low levels also induce impulsive behavior and the compulsion for immediate gratification.

With high levels, both males and females tend to orgasm more quickly, although sex drive is somewhat blunted. When dieting, serotonin levels diminish, which may account for the sexy feeling we get when we shed a few pounds.

Dopamine controls the desire or drive for pleasure, both sexual and otherwise. With dopamine, we feel elated and excited. When levels of this neurotransmitter are low, we feel flat and feel no joy, pleasure, or enthusiasm. Dopamine is the common denominator in all addictions. It may also be what addicts us to each other, since it promotes anticipation of pleasure and sex drive. Dopamine intensifies our experiences. It makes us want to have them over and over again. It motivates us to seek pleasure.

Progesterone is the killer of sex drive. It does so by reducing sex drive in both sexes. It also reduces pheromones and can make us smell bad to the other species. It makes women irritable towards men and aggressive. The irritable aggressive nature is a way for the female of the species to protect the young against the male of the species. Many animals eat the young because they are easy prey, so the female becomes aggressive and protective by progesterone. And yet progesterone also makes females nurturing towards their young.

Prolactin is a gentle hormone that increases with pregnancy and nursing. It diminishes sex drive. When men develop high levels of prolactin they lose their sex drive and become impotent. Dopamine prohibits prolactin, thereby increasing sex drive, whereas estrogen gradually increases with prolactin secretion, diminishing the aggressive sex drive and leaving women with the receptive drive of estrogen.

Finally, vasopressin, the "monogamy molecule." Vasopressin works closely with testosterone, keeping it from reaching extremes of aggression. Vasopressin tempers us and is somewhat dulling and stabilizing. It governs human temperature and keeps one's temper from raging out of control. However, it also mutes the intensity of certain feelings, making our emotional range somewhat narrow. It turns our attention away from the abstract and into the concrete; away from the past and the future and into the present moment. It seems to improve memory, cognitive powers, and concentration. Therefore, it is an advantage when it comes to focus and pleasure in lovemaking. It is the molecule that encourages us to create and stay in monogamous relationship. It is the emotional glue that binds us together.

These are the key players when it comes to sex drive, love, and emotions. There are a host of other players that also influence life's pleasures and delights; but for simplicity's sake, we will focus on this cast of players.

Like the ebb and flow of the tides, our hormones and peptides fluctuate throughout the hour, the day, the month, and our entire lives. Many factors influence the release and contraction of these biochemical substances. In the following pages we will examine some of the natural things we can do to enhance and enjoy our sexual being, because after all; first in life, through life, and after life (the afterlife you ask? spiritual eternity perhaps or on the death certificate it will eternally be) you are a sexual being.

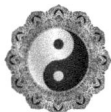

~ A successful life: to find and experience true love. ~

WHAT HAPPENED?
THE THRILL IS GONE

For this chapter, I conducted an independent research project. I randomly interviewed people I did not know about their marriages and relationships. I wanted to know why the fires of passion burn out, and although the circumstances may differ, the underlying reasons were clear. Let us see if we can walk through the nature of relationships.

Chemistry and attraction — what is it that draws two people together? Why is it that you can meet a variety of people and the percentage that you find attractive is so small and even smaller is the percentage that exudes chemistry. We all know it when we feel it, but lack the understanding of how to find it at will. It is just one of those things that happens. You can date hundreds of people before you feel it, and then suddenly, out of the blue, there it is smack in your face, the illusive spark of chemistry. Your head spins, your knees buckle, your heart pounds, and your stomach is full of fluttering butterflies. You are suddenly lust struck!

We can see a person and find them sexy and attractive but the chemistry is not there, and we can see someone who is not conventionally good-looking and sexy and they drive us crazy with the chemistry of lust. What is the magic that makes two people feel that spark at the same time and with the same intensity?

In the last chapter, we looked at hormones and neurochemicals that rush through the body and drive us to mate but that does not explain the chemistry between two people. Ever looked at a couple and wondered what they see in each other? It is chemistry of a unique kind. Yes, it is driven by the biochemistry of our being, but it is not the biological drive alone. It is something more that brings two people together.

Although we can explain it through biochemistry we cannot explain, dictate, arrange, or make it happen at will. There is something mysterious and fatalistic about finding that person who "floats your boat."

The strange thing about mutual chemistry is that, although it does not happen often in life, it does happen more than once. We can "fall in love" more than once in our lifetime. The problem is that this "falling in love" stage is usually the result of hormones rushing through our being, creating a euphoric rush that leaves little room for rational thought. We simply get lost in the flood of chemistry and lose sight of the long-term relationship.

However, if it were not for this act of nature we would never come together and procreate. It is the animalistic biological urge to mate, combined with the human urge to find love that is the driving force behind mating, pairing, and monogamy. If only it was this simple. Many factors come into play once the rush of chemistry subsides and the reality of long-term mating and loving set in. This is when the nature of relationships changes.

So what happens as we go from lust to love and then to "the thrill is gone"? It all begins with the chemistry of lust. We see someone across a crowded room and suddenly we are lustfully excited. The dopamine rushes through our brain. We get high and giddy. The pleasure center ignites, and we feel on top of the world. Life gets exciting. We feel that surge of attraction. It is such a heady feeling that we will abandon our family, jobs, money, and time for a moment of stolen pleasure. We are willing to risk security and disease for that lustful moment of pure delight.

We get excited again about life. Suddenly we are at the gym, eating healthfully, grooming, and caring about being sexy and alluring. We whistle, laugh, sing, and renew our enthusiasm for other pleasures in life like art, music, dance, and hobbies of all sorts. Creativity is enhanced as our new muse offers up excitement. We get high on dopamine and will rearrange almost everything in our lives to be with the person of our desire.

The sexual fires begin to burn as the testosterone and estrogen play out the dance of sex. All our sexual pistons are firing and all we can think about is mating. It is the challenge and the chase that keeps the urge strong. If the chemistry lasts beyond the initial attraction, we begin the dance of romance.

Romance is different from initial physical attraction. Now we want more. We want to know the person. We are fascinated with every story and every nuance of this person. Everything seems right. We are filled with butterflies at the very sight of our lover, and all we know is that we want more.

Therefore, we put our best foot forward and begin to romance the other in an attempt to find love. We want this to be the one. We want to be in love and we are sure this must be the one because we feel so warm and squishy inside. This has to be true love. It does not come along every day so we make every effort to make it work.

Flowers, perfume, sexy clothes, fancy dinners, escapes to resorts, gifts, backrubs, and plenty of sex.

Then we fall in love, determined to spend the rest of our lives with our lover. "This must be it," we tell ourselves. This is what love feels like, and this time it will last forever. And despite what well-meaning friends and family may tell us, we cannot see any faults or any problems. The other person is perfect. Our relationship is perfect. Others do not understand the depth of our love. We are going to spend the rest of our lives together in loving, sensual, and sexual bliss.

So we plan to make it official, and we decide to get married. But first, we'll live together because that's what people do these days. So we move in, rearrange our lives to fit the new us, and prepare ourselves for continual sex, love, pleasure, and joy. And then the first real fight happens. The bubble bursts and suddenly we are vulnerable and hurt. How could this happen? We are in love!

So we both back down and give in because we want to get back to the sex and the pleasure of being in love. The romance and love is still so new and still so full of chemically charged hormones and emotionally charged feelings of pleasure. The makeup sex is great and we fall back in love again...until the next time. And there *will* be a next time. Because once the reality of life begins to set in — dirty laundry, morning breath, moods, issues, and stress — arguments arise and the relationship must be negotiated. But not until we are married! So we get caught up in the rush of wedding plans and the joy of a blissful life of love forever after.

After the marriage, the honeymoon phase sets in. We believe that marriage is the end of our problems and will bring us a life of happiness, fulfillment, togetherness, and joy. It is supposed to end the loneliness and the fear of not finding our true love. In the honeymoon phase, we fight and tug at the edges of our relationship as we try to adjust to married life. In this phase, we are still in love, and the fighting usually returns to makeup sex and back to blissful intimacy. However, this phase is short-lived.

Statistics tell us sex usually dwindles to about once a week after the first year of marriage. From a survey conducted since 1972 by the data from General Social Survey, the average happily married couple has sex about 58 times a year. Those couples under thirty average about 111 times a year. They define a sexless marriage (relationship) as having sex 10 or fewer times a year. Fifteen percent of married couples have had no sex in the last six months. How could this happen and what does this mean?

There are so many factors that influence one's sexual life and far too many choices to describe all the possibilities. We could start with a few of the things that can affect a relationship: attraction, mistrust, children, hurt, excuses, sickness, stress, tired, asexual, low sex drive, been abused, taken for granted, gay (and not wanting to admit it), financial, infidelity, secrets, desires, the choice of one's partner, children, family; just to mention the most obvious influences that can make a relationship get shaky. Now couple any or all of the above with the biochemical changes that come with age, poor diet, and lack of exercise and we can see how easily our sex lives are affected.

Although many factors can be involved, it is up to you to discover and enhance your own sexuality. Removing negatives, barriers, and dishonesty are part of the secret to a healthier sex life. Therefore, it would be fair to say that our sex life has to do with a host of things, which all boil down to the body, the mind, and the soul. When we seek to balance and focus the so-called three vehicles of being, a gateway opens and dissolves negatives, barriers, and dishonesty. Nature provides many opportunities to nurture and feed the body, mind, and soul towards sexual enhancement.

To fully understand what happened and why the passion, the romance, the sensuality, and the sexuality has dwindled, one only needs to look to one's self and decide to focus on improving one's sexual health. This path is not easy, but once chosen, it may lead you to the aphrodisiac of life. Think about how great you felt when you were in love: sexy, passionate, loving, kind, close, caring, vital, sharp, vigorous, strong, and playful with a touch of flirtatious charm. When you create this within yourself, the doors to renewed passion will open and you will experience the aphrodisiac of life.

Ask yourself these questions:
Do I want to renew my sexual passions with my current partner?
Am I looking to reconnect sexually?
Do I want to feel sexy, happy, healthy, and alive?

If you cannot do it with the person you are with because you are not attracted to that person and do not love that person, then you should move on. Because being dishonest about love and attraction hurts you the most. Never has dishonesty been an attractive trait. If you want to feel sexy and alive and the person you love has abandoned you, then get yourself sexually healthy; and if they do not take notice and want to join, move on and find someone who will. Be kind to yourself and develop your own self-esteem along with a deep understanding of what it takes to make life a sensual experience.

While researching this subject, I read something interesting on askmen.com. The author was discussing the reasons that women stop having sex after marriage and how difficult it is on men. He concluded it wisely:

Ludwig Borne put it best when he said,
"A sweetheart is milk, a bride is butter and a wife is cheese."

Now, before everyone sends hate mail and death threats, let me add that my theory applies to both genders. To a woman a boyfriend is like wine, a groom is like cocktails, and a husband is like flat beer. After all, the definition of love, philosophically speaking, is attraction preceded by admiration.

In addition, I would add that a woman can stay a sweetheart and a man can remain a boyfriend, even years into a marriage. If either one or both should slip from that place, there is always a way to get back there. It takes a little work combined with a little admiration and appreciation and the attraction will return.

One of my favorite books on love is a book by Sol Gordon, Ph.D., *How Can You Tell if You're Really in Love?* One of the reasons I love this book is that Dr. Gordon gives us permission to feel revenge. We all know the feeling of anger, disappointment, sadness, and hurt should love dwindle. Nevertheless, we are told it is bad to want to seek out revenge. Dr. Gordon puts it this way: "it is okay to want to seek revenge. The best revenge is taken when you choose to live well and take care of yourself. Nothing will move you past a disappointing love affair faster than feeling good about yourself by living healthy and well. It is one of life's little sexual secrets."

Resentment, anger, and disappointment will change a relationship from one of love to one of destruction. I believe that underneath all fading romance is the disappointment that comes from discovering that the person we are with and the relationship we are in does not meet our expectations. Of course, if one marries for money, social status, to end loneliness, out of desperation, or because our family will accept the person, then we cannot complain when the sexual and romantic flames fade. For sensual pleasure to endure there must be the spark of attraction. Moreover, from this spark of attraction, there must be a foundation of love, trust, and respect to reignite the passionate fires.

When one partner falls out of love with the other, an intimate relationship is doomed. It is very difficult to be intimate with someone you do not love and maybe cannot stand. When this happens, it is very painful for the man or woman who still is in love and still wants to make the relationship work. When continuing arguments happen, no one wants to be loving and sexual. This leads to feelings of being deprived, resentful, and angry. One partner (usually the husband) will accuse the other of being sexually uninterested, which is not necessarily true. The person is sexually interested, but not with their partner. The relationship then begins to slip away and a divorce ensues or they decide to live a rather passionless and empty relationship. Over and over through my research, I heard this story. People married for over 10 years (average about 15 years) find themselves not attracted to their mate.

It can range from any set of circumstances. The fires have died and neither wants to put forth the effort to make it work. So they go about their daily lives, each living in a silence of loneliness.

This is the stuff of affairs. Most people, due to children and money, do not want to go through a divorce so they seek out affairs, hoping the thrill of the new person and the intimate encounter will bring excitement and pleasure without a cost to anyone. Nevertheless, I would contend that never has an affair been without cost. Even if no one ever finds out, the affair has an effect on the marriage that will be destructive. Dishonesty and mistrust will always be present.

Affairs happen because something is missing. When something is missing and we seek to replace it through dishonest means, respect is lost. When we create something new through an affair, we break something old, which is the bond and commitment of a relationship. Now if both parties openly agree to stay together and look the other way at indiscretion, then all is open, and if it works, there has been a respect for each other.

When I interviewed people for this book, everyone who was looking for an affair or in an affair told me that the passion was gone, the intimacy was null, and the sex was less than 10 times a year. Everyone felt lonely and deprived. One man I met was married to a woman who had put on a lot of weight and was suffering from depression. She felt so bad about herself that she turned cold to her husband. She refused to have sex with him. He felt deprived and lonely. He was in his early 50s and still wanted to have a sex life. He told me that he felt he had a right to have an affair without telling her, because she was denying him the intimacy and sex that he desired. He told me that if she were warm and loving the excess weight would be okay.

He tried to talk with her but she just pushed him away. When I met him, he was onto his third affair. He was a professional by now, and knew how to cover up and not be caught. He was way beyond guilt. As he told me, he had crossed to the other side and could now conduct his affairs and receive the pleasure he deserved. This, he told me, was not what he expected would happen to his marriage. However, he had been married before and had experienced the same thing. His ex-wife had shut down so he concluded that all women shut down, so it was better to stay and get the benefits of marriage and then have affairs. In life, we can justify anything!

Over and over I heard the same story. The relationship was fine. They did not fight. Children and money kept them together. The passion was gone and the sex was gone. They were living like brother and sister. They traveled and on occasion had sex but intimacy, play, laughter, and that deep passionate spark was gone. Maybe it was never there and maybe they picked the wrong person. The thrill was gone, and over and over each person longed to feel the thrill of passion and lust. They craved the excitement of sexual newness and attraction. They obsessed over the high ride of sexual chemistry. They wanted the thrill again and again.

Why was the thrill gone? Why did it slip away? Was it really ever there?

It begins with a deep attraction and understanding of the other person. It also means we take care of ourselves. We keep active and we grow. We stay interesting and sexy. We care enough about ourselves and the intimacy of love to work hard and keep the relationship healthy and alive.

The initial thrill of attraction is short-lived. We all crave it and miss it when it is gone, but it is the wise person who realizes that in every relationship the thrill will come and go and that every relationship brings its own host of problems, decisions, joys, disappointments, and surprises. The grass may look greener on the other side but from the other side it is the same green grass.

Current data about Americans reveal that 85 percent marry and about 60 percent divorce. Of those 60 percent, 75 percent remarry and almost 50 percent of these marriages fail. Why do they fail? Because we fail to look at the package deal when choosing a partner. We marry for the love, lifestyle, and compatibility but fail to look at the character of the person and to realize that with time all things change. It is hard work to make a relationship last. Yes, a relationship can last years without passion or sex but when the thrill is gone, life takes on a dull and lackluster sheen.

Dr. Gordon writes about the three essential ingredients to making a relationship last:

- Sense of humor
- Wisdom to overlook a lot of stuff
- A basic respect for each other no matter what

He poses the question: *without these three things would it matter how attractive a person was? How good would sex be with a humorless sourpuss who obsesses over every little thing you do and has no respect for you?*

If you find yourself wanting to reignite the sparks of sexual energy and your partner is willing, then read along and follow this book. If your partner is not willing, do it on your own and you might be surprised when your partner takes notice and wants to join. If your partner is done, or you are done or you are alone, looking for a new partner; then do it for yourself and watch what happens when you reignite your own passion. Something exciting might happen!

So now, let us recap:

The thrill dissipates for a variety of reasons. If the attraction was not there to begin with, then any attempt to make it hot will quickly die. Children, stress, money, family life, work, incompatibilities, anger, hurt, sexual drives, letting your appearance go, disinterest, abuse, alcohol, drugs, gambling, infidelity, fighting, trust, and all the other negatives of life can destroy intimacy. When the thrill is gone and not replaced with affection, love, respect, caring, and deep devotion, wandering will happen.

In my research talking with random men and women who are looking for affairs, this is what I discovered:

On average, somewhere between 10 and 15 years into a relationship, one or both partners will have an affair. This first affair is usually short-lived and comes as a surprise. Someone walks into your life, you are feeling unhappy and lonely, and you take the plunge. Mostly, it happens to men. Women are very busy at this point with the children and the home and may not have the opportunity that men have in the working world. Restlessness and the need for attention is usually the cause, but just because a woman is home does not mean she would not like to have the same opportunity.

Things usually settle down for a while, although most people are open to another affair should the opportunity arise. Somewhere around 20 years the itch reappears. This seems to be a magical number for seeking out an affair. Almost everyone I surveyed who was looking for an affair had been married between 18 and 22 years. Compellingly, the reasons were mostly the same. The thrill was gone, the passion was null and void, and they were longing for that feeling of excitement, the adrenaline rush and dopamine fix that comes from the physical attraction of lust. Without a doubt, no one was looking to leave their marriage and most stated that their marriage was good but the sex was either gone or almost gone, and they just didn't talk any more. The reasons for staying were money and children. Everyone seemed to think that an affair might be good for the marriage. It might give them the missing piece in their life while remaining married. No one gets hurt, and they get to relive their sexual and sensual passion before it is too late. It was never about the sex. It was always about the need for affection and passion. Loneliness was the biggest factor.

When I asked how they would feel if their spouse had an affair, almost without thought each person would recoil into himself or herself and quickly dismiss the idea. It seems its okay for the goose but not for the gander or vice versa!

So we get married and enter into wedded bliss. Along the way we hurt each other, discover each other's inadequacies, have children, buy homes, work hard, deal with stress, grow older, become complacent, stop relating, the sex dwindles, the fires die, passion is killed, and the thrill is gone.

Now the good news is that almost everyone I spoke with, both men and women, loved their mates, and would love it if the sex, passion, and lovemaking could return. They all said they would not be cheating if the play, sex, fun, and affection were present in their marriage. They would be more than willing to find the thrill again but had no idea how to rekindle the home fires.

Something was missing. A void existed. Everyone felt loneliness and boredom. Everyone wanted something more, but no one wanted to give up the comforts of their marriage, including the money, home, and the children.

When the thrill is gone, you can look everywhere to find it again, but essentially, it begins with you. What you put back into your relationship is exactly what you will get from it. If you make an effort to romance your partner and work to reignite the fires of passion then either your partner will respond in kind or ignore your overtures. If you are rejected and you have sincerely tried, you will not lose. By reigniting your own sexual health and energy, you will naturally draw to yourself exciting and interesting people, places, and things. If your partner chooses to stay complacent then you will know you have done your best. And with this, you may find the courage to be honest because honesty is still the best policy. An affair hurts everyone and eventually everyone finds out. Dishonesty has never been a sexually attractive trait. This is not to take the moral high ground but when we cheat on others, we must be prepared to be cheated on. If we enter into a marriage with a commitment to be honest, respectful, and trustworthy, cheating defies all our commitments. If we enter into a relationship with no commitments or expectations, then judgment is suspended. However, if we make promises either overtly or as a general understanding and cannot keep those promises, isn't it best to be open and honest?

Sexual health is more than excitement, thrills, and orgasms. It is an energetic feeling dressed in charisma, laughter, and play. It is about the body, mind, and soul united. When we are sexually healthy, we draw creative energy to ourselves. We love and care for others in deep and meaningful ways.

Sexual infidelity has been a remedy for sexual health and excitement since the beginning of time. Affairs happen and will continue to happen. The question to ask yourself is, am I okay with "Do unto others, as I would have them do unto me"?

I would dare to say that everyone in a long-term relationship gets bored and restless from time to time. Most likely, everyone thinks about a passing affair. It is human nature to want the thrill of lust and love over and over again. What seems to stop a person from having an affair is the fear of being caught and losing the person they truly love. When you love and respect a person, you do not want to hurt them. The depth of true love overrides the temporary rush of lustful passion.

So now, rather than dwell on the thrill, the lust, and the reasons for infidelity, let's move forward and focus on how to enhance and support our sexual health.

By focusing on your sexual health, you will feel sexier, happier, and recapture that radiance, vim, and vigor of your most creative and passionate self. You will experience that magical place called ecstasy. If you are in a relationship, ask your partner to come along and enjoy the fun. If they refuse, do it for you and watch the magic unfold. If you are alone and searching for a love partner, enhance your sexual self, and before you know it, you'll be drawing into your life other sexually charged and exciting people.

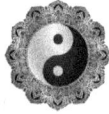

~ So what exactly is sexual health? ~

IT'S A NATURAL THING

S exuality is a natural thing. It is the very vein of creation. No matter what your orientation it is a fundamental aspect of being human. There have been times throughout history where sex has been treated as something forbidden, sordid, shameful, and vulgar. Groups and institutions have tried to control the expression of our sexual nature. The desire to have sex or the expression of sex is so strong that it has the ability to literally change or transmute one form of energy into another. Generally speaking, we associate the energy of sex with the physical. However, the desire of sexual expression has behind it the potential of perpetuating humankind, maintaining health (it is a proven scientific fact that a healthy sex life improves general overall health), and the creative expression that transforms mediocrity into genius.

Sex is such a powerful drive that humans will risk their lives, families, and fortunes to indulge in it. When harnessed and redirected toward creative endeavors, this powerful motivating force enhances literature, art, and any other creative calling, including the accumulation of wealth. Sex is a powerful drive that can be transformed into dynamic energy.

However, this transformation of sex energy from the physical lustful aspect to creative expression requires will power. The desire for sexual expression is inborn and natural. It should not be submerged or discouraged but rather allowed to express itself freely through creative outlets that enrich the body, mind, and soul of humankind. The very nature of sex is to seek expression. Give it a creative outlet, and what will emerge are excitement, joy, and ultimate pleasure.

Fortunate is the person who has learned how to nourish this creative expression. Biographies have taught us that both men and women with highly developed sex natures have achieved great heights. Charisma and vital energy has always been a sexual draw, and behind each charismatic person is usually a lover, confidant, and greatest supporter. Why? Because healthy sexual expression encompasses more than the physical act. It involves body, mind, and soul harmoniously blending into a balanced, centered being.

The study of naturopathy is about teaching the general philosophy that we are tri-part beings — body, mind, and soul — and it is the balancing of all three states of being that brings about perfect health. If the body is healthy and strong and the mind is sharp and clear so that the body-mind can unite with the soul and touch that place of appreciation, contemplation,

gratitude, peace, and happiness, you have perfect health. Everything is in perfect balance. Diet, exercise, herbs, essentials oils, color/light, music, and meditation and contemplation are used to balance health.

Your sexuality is your body, mind, and soul. Why wouldn't you want to balance it out and reclaim that vivacious and delicious self? It is natural to want it and natural to get it. We simply need to look at the whole rather than individual pieces. After all, the one thing you carry with you your entire life is your sexuality. It is with you no matter what — it's a very big part in defining your life. Therefore, the most important thing in our lives is our health. I like to quote a writing attributed to Herophiles, 300 B.C., a physician who was an early performer of public dissection on human cadavers and often called the father of anatomy:

"When health is absent, wisdom cannot reveal itself, art cannot become manifest, strength cannot be exerted, wealth is useless, and reason is powerless."

Therefore, to have one's health provides the ability to find wisdom, express your creative endeavor, be vital, have the potential to gain wealth, and the ability to reason. So sex and health are, as they say, "like hand to glove." One without the other is a sad and lonely place. From a naturopathic standpoint, the best way to ensure a healthy sexual self is through using the methods employed by naturopathy, which is to balance the energy of the body, mind, and soul. Keeping your sexual health is fundamental to a life that experiences passion, joy, and pleasure.

Remember, sex is a natural thing. Healthy adults well into their 70s and beyond still participate in sexual activity. It is as natural as eating, drinking, working, and playing. In other words, it is a natural part of everyday life.

Although in our youth we take it for granted, sex is a phenomenal part of our happiness beyond the mere act, the orgasm, and procreation. Sex influences our lives is so many ways. Ask anyone in a relationship, and he or she will tell you that sex is important. It defines the relationship, not only physically, but also mentally and spiritually.

Psychologically speaking sexuality refers to the reproductive and erotic dimensions of human life. Freudian psychology was perhaps the dominant force in shaping modern perspectives on sexuality, exerting an influence that extended well beyond the audience of academic and professional psychologists. Freud treated sexuality as the force behind the formation of the psyche and nearly all subsequent adult behavior. Any deviance from what was termed "normal" sex was seen as a psychological disorder. Today we view sexuality much differently. We know that people have different orientations and different drives. This is not to say that one's sexual outlook does not have a basis in experience, both negative and positive. Incest, rape, and other factors can severely damage a healthy sex life.

For the purposes of this book, we are looking only at the health of the human being and how a healthy approach to sexuality through natural methods can enhance both our sex life and the vitality and creativity of the individual. Sex is not only about procreation, nor is it simply about recreation. In a balanced sense, it is about a healthy approach to living one's life.

So let us look at what natural health is all about. What exactly is the study of naturopathy, and what does it have to do with a healthy and natural sex life? Balance is the essence of a healthy life. Sex is natural. It has the potential to bring balanced health into your life. However, it must be approached from a healthy perspective, which includes fun and play.

In yoga, there is a fundamental philosophy that we should seek balance in all things and in all things find balance. This means all things in moderation. We need to dispel the words good and bad and replace them with a focus on bringing into our lives those things that bring balance in body, mind, and spirit.

When someone comes to a naturopath with issues of depression, low energy, and restlessness, we first look at the biochemistry of the body. Nutrition, we know, affects our moods, energy levels, hormones, and the overall chemistry of our body. So we need to teach the individual about good health through a healthy diet and exercise. These are the two underpinnings of natural health. Hippocrates, the father of modern medicine, said, "Let foods be our medicine."

From the time of Hippocrates, it has been well documented that certain food has life-giving properties. Healthy whole natural foods have the power to heal and to prevent disease. Despite all this documentation, humans are fast approaching an epidemic of obesity, diabetes, heart disease, and other maladies associated with poor eating habits.

Prescription medicine is a bandage approach to stabilizing disease. Sometimes, we need to use allopathic medicine to bring about stabilization. The problem begins when we do not take it a step further and apply the principles of a healthy lifestyle to bring about balanced health. No therapy or drug known to humankind can rebuild tissue that has been damaged by disease or trauma. Only healthy food gives us the fuel that rebuilds and rejuvenates the human body.

Good nutrition is not simply about physical health; it is about life enrichment and well-being. Sadly, many people are not living up to their vital potential due to poor diet and lack of exercise. The same foods that help to build new tissue also help to enhance wellness by increasing the efficiency and energy levels of organs, glands, and tissues such as the skin, muscles, joints, nerves, veins, and arteries. Simply put: you can enhance your health and experience vitality through eating a healthy diet.

Exercise is scientifically proven to enhance health. Next to nutrition, exercise is the most important natural thing we can do for our health. Exercise gives back energy, vitality, vigor, and vim. Exercise is a proven sexual enhancer. Science tells us that regular exercise is good for the heart, blood pressure, weight control, immunity boosting , bone building , flexibility, balance, strength, and aerobic capacity, as well as hormonal and biochemical release such as endorphins.

Endorphins are a class of neurotransmitters that the brain produces. Endorphins act as a break on pain and then most likely transfer that pain to a feeling of well-being. When the body is stressed, such as during exercise, we call this release of endorphins a "runner's high."

It works like this: Endorphin synapses in the brain inhibit neurons that produce GABA.

GABA functions as a neurotransmitter in the central nervous system by decreasing neuron activity and thereby bringing a calm and tranquil feeling to the body-mind. Exercise produces endorphins, which prohibit neurons that prohibit the release of GABA. This inhibition of inhibition increases dopamine, which is the neurotransmitter that is released when we feel sexually turned on.

Here's how it works: every cell in the body builds some of the material it needs by chemical reactions on ingested substances found in the diet to produce the chemicals necessary for normal functioning. The neuron is no exception. Our diet and exercise have profound effects on the nature of our being. Our general overall health — and specifically for the purpose of this book, our sexual health — depends upon balancing out the biochemistry of existence through natural means like diet and exercise.

Naturopathy also addresses the balancing of the mind, thoughts, and consciousness. Diet and exercise as well as other natural methods (herbs, oils, music, etc.) will help to bring balance to the mind through the release of neurochemicals that stabilize the nutritional health of the body. However, if the mind does not resolve its imbalances (emotions), it will be very difficult to stay on the healthy path because the mind loses its focus and energy gets out of balance. In naturopathy, we try first to address issues of depression, anxiety, low energy, or whatever malady the individual should bring to a session, with proper teaching about nutrition. Nevertheless, we must also help the person to find psychological balance. We do not practice psychotherapy, but rather spend time talking with an individual about stressors, problems, needs, and desires.

The quest, then, is to help the individual find a place within the mind where there is a sense of calm, focus, and a change in perspective and attitude. It is not about having positive thoughts because just trying to have positive

thoughts does not alleviate the issue of a scattered and imbalanced mind. It means to get to a place where we look at things neither as good nor bad but simply phenomena in our lives that have many dimensions. There are many ways to look at the same thing. When looked at from a balanced and focused point of view, problems are solvable and decisions are easily made because, after all, what is the nature of life but problems to solve and decisions to be made?

A naturopath can only guide and teach you along the path the naturopath has taken. The path is presented as a possibility and the choice is entirely up to you. Clearing and uplifting the mind certainly makes way for a happier and healthier life. The mind is a vibrating energetic mechanism that allows you to create thoughts. Thoughts given energy have the power to accomplish any goal.

I have combined my yoga teaching with naturopathy to help individuals reach a place of quiet mind. It is a method of simply stopping and taking a deep breath, being in the moment, experiencing the moment, as the moment should be...quiet and calm. Oftentimes, it is this quieting of the mind that precedes focusing on nutrition and the balancing of the energy of the body.

I have used Bach Flower Remedies® and aromatherapy to help open up the thought channels of a person's mind. Often there is blockage that needs to be released. With a quiet approach, using herbs, light, color, aromatherapy, and soft music, the perspective often changes. It may change for only short amounts of time, but if the individual continues to apply these tools, the transformation will take place.

For example, if a person were depressed, Bach would recommend wild rose as an elixir to help one realize that it is necessary to change one's negative mental programming. Bach believed that "There is no true healing unless there is a change in outlook, peace of mind, and inner happiness."

I would then bring out an essential oil (such as jasmine or ylang-ylang) for its uplifting and sensual properties. The scent of a euphoric essential oil just like the wonderful scent of a flower is sure to assist one out of a state of sadness and depression.

Now let us move onto the third part of our being, the spirit or the soul.

It is essential to bring peace and balance to the soul. The soul is that restless and impatient side of you. It is full of passion and energy. It is how you direct the energy of your being that determines the essence of your life. Here, I would recommend meditation and contemplation: a time-out to sit quietly and find the essence beneath the layers of energy known as the *sheath*. Some might understand this as the aura, which I will talk about later in the book when we get to color and light vibrations.

Now, there may be some of you questioning the existence of a soul. You may think that it is your mind that is the essence of being or that we are simply a body-mind driven by instincts and biology. I would ask you to look at your own inner world behind the thoughts and feel the energy known as self.

It has been said that when needed there is a driven spirit within humans that is capable of extreme feats. The spirit of humankind comes forth in times of disaster. It is a force beyond mental reason and physical strength.

The spirit captures those few moments in time where we are awestruck by what we perceive to be beauty. Each person has his or her own definition of beauty and unique experience when encountering it. This is the soul's energy.

However, the soul is not selfish and overbearing. It sits back and waits for the body-mind to find a space where it can be heard. When the body-mind is thrashing about it is somewhat difficult to experience beauty. The soul's energy is best experienced in the place where subconsciousness and consciousness meet and consciousness begins to unfold. You will know it when you experience a momentary transcendence from the body-mind much like the ecstasy of an orgasm.

The law of karma, which is purification, means action. It means the total universe in action where everything is dynamically connected with everything else. To transcend karma is to keep going into the gap, which is the place between your earthly persona and your soul. Each time you experience the gap you have the opportunity to get closer to your soul. To transcend this is to go beyond action and consequence and begin to make conscious choices. You are then no longer controlled by karma but make conscious choices that are evolutionary for you and those around you.

This brings us to our witnessing consciousness. This is where we are able to step back from ourselves and witness our actions consciously. We choose rather than react to circumstances. This implies nonjudgmental behavior. When you are constantly judging things as good or bad you create turmoil in the body-mind. This turmoil restricts the flow of energy between you and your higher self and thus blocks the way to your potentiality.

The greatest challenge for us is maintaining our spiritual connection every day and living by it. It is just like a physical fitness program. To stay physically fit you need to get up every day and make the choice to exercise. Those who are committed to keeping themselves physically fit never belabor over the choice but simply make exercise a part of their daily routine. It is the same way with the foods that we eat and the thoughts we keep. Consciously and unconsciously we make choices in each moment of how we choose to live our lives. This is the voice of the ego, which constantly challenges the spirit. When the spirit and the ego blend, a softening occurs and we experience a moment of ecstasy.

We will discuss the role of the spiritual self in attaining sexual health later on in this book. For now, it is important to remember that we are body, mind, and soul and the balancing of all three together brings about perfect health.

Any assessment of health must be looked at from the perspective of body, mind, soul, environment, relationships, and food. Imbalance or sickness in any of these areas will be reflected to some degree in the others.

The foundation of natural healing is summarized in the statement *"All healing comes from within, and the body-mind heals itself."* Therefore, before any true healing can take place we must be willing to look at the true cause of our illness on all levels: body, mind, and soul. We must be willing to surrender to our deepest wisdom, which is the seat of our soul, and implement whatever methods will bring our entire being back into balance. It is a mistake to implement any form of healing or health regimen without recognizing the need to acknowledge the above and be willing to surrender.

Allopathic drugs with their sometimes-deadly side effects may bring quick and temporary relief from pain but they do nothing to restore and rejuvenate the body. They may, in fact — as in the case of antibiotics — leave the body weaker. Even natural remedies such as diet, herbs, and exercise may not be appropriate without the right healing attitude. This proper attitude is the ability to see our problems from a broader perspective as a process of readjustment or a valuable lesson to be learned.

Our lives are ever flowing, waning and waxing like the moon. Obstacles present themselves and teach us. It is the resistance to this flow of life that is the primary cause of all our suffering. Life is about change and learning to flow with the energy of change. This is the process of evolution of which we are an intricate part. Illness, depression, and misfortune are simply messages informing us of imbalances and providing a guidepost for discovering the negative energies that we have cultivated. Awareness of and correcting the negative qualities is the path to spiritual fitness and thus physical and mental fitness. Bad diets, weight problems, illness, depression, addiction, accidents, and self-neglect are simply a reflection of our disconnection with our spiritual being. Enduring changes intended to remove an unhealthy diet, promote exercise, and remove stress must be accompanied by spiritual realization if true growth and health are to occur. The process of change is seen as a process of awakening to a new life.

Therefore, the key factor of natural health is balance. But balance is sometimes so difficult for us to attain. It seems boring and lacks the passion and the excitement of pushing the envelope and tasting the richness of life. But this is not necessarily true.

Living natural for many of us is so far removed from our lifestyles that we have forgotten what things really taste like, smell like, and feel like. Our taste buds and sense of smell have been corrupted by a synthetic world.

Proportion means only enough to satisfy a need. Needs and wants differ. In our society, we always want more. We no longer eat or consume to satisfy a need (life-health) but consume on all levels to satisfy our want to have more! Bigger, faster, and more is supposed to bring us happiness and fulfillment. Sadly, this mass consumption is the result of feeling incomplete and does not bring happiness. A balanced diet combined with exercise moves us from outward consumption to inner fulfillment.

Although we all know we should do some form of exercise each day, it is easy to make exercise low on the priority list. After all, it takes time and effort and we have so many other important things to do. It's all about attitude and priorities.

Probably the most difficult thing to change is our attitude. Attitudes are framed around beliefs and become intrinsic parts of our personality. The balance is sometimes unclear.

Health and fitness in the body-mind make it easy to open the doorway to the spiritual self. This is because one is not weighed down by layers of earthly pollution such as obesity, addictions, and poor physical and mental health. Balance is always found through the choices we make.

To stay physically fit you need to get up every day and make the choice to exercise. Remember those who are committed to keeping themselves physically fit *never belabor the choice* but simply make exercise a part of their daily routine. It is the same way with the foods that we eat and the thoughts we keep. Consciously and unconsciously we choose each moment of how we live our lives. It is the voice of the ego, which constantly challenges the spirit in an attempt to throw us off balance.

Without balancing and integrating all aspects of self, we miss the territory for the map. Honoring the body-mind, we set about to give the best care to that royal chariot, you, that sets us about on our earthly journey. Spiritual fitness then becomes a way of life where honor and devotion is given to self and the entire universe. As the Buddha said, *once you are on the spiritual path you cannot help but live a healthy life.*

Sexual health is body, mind, and soul connected at its core. When we naturally support the health of our sexual self, excitement, passion, and enrichment spring forth with great intensity. When passion exists and excitement is strong, and it comes from a place of balance, I can promise you, life is not boring!

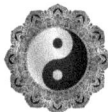

*~ Now let's take a closer look at the natural methods
used to enhance your sexual health. ~*

APHRODISIACS

N o doubt, we have all heard of Aphrodite, the Greek goddess of love and beauty. The word *aphrodisiac* is derived from the legend of Aphrodite's magic potions. Aphrodisiacs are potions that are said to arouse sexual desire. The nature of human attraction and relationships has perplexed humans since the beginning of time. We search for elixirs and magic potions in the hope that they will bring to us the object of our desire. Tales of love, lust, and romance have been a part of the whole mystical process.

The Greeks and the Romans were masters at the art of romantic myths. A myth is defined as the talking or retelling of a story. Most are fables and folktales without historic verification. They are based upon stories of animals and real humans. A second kind of myth was that of a saga or legend. The difference was that a saga or legend was about people, gods, and monsters. Sagas were based upon actual characters and events, such as the famous *Iliad*, the epic story of a phase of the Trojan War. A third type of myth is referred to as pure or true myth. These are stories about the origins and development of religions and rituals. Some anthropologists believe that the emergence of some form of ritual was the defining creation of human culture. Greek mythology made verse to youth, sex, and physical perfection through the tales of Zeus, who lusted after earthly women; Cupid and Psyche (whose name means soul), the god and the mortal who fell in love and found each other; Pygmalion and Galatea, the sculptor who fell in love with his statue of the perfect woman; and Pomona and Vertumnus, who forever appeared strong and youthful. All of these myths were tales of beauty, lust, and love.

One thing all these myths had in common is that they dealt with gods and their interactions with human beings. What made Greeks and Romans different was that much of their mythology was based upon the gods having human form and even human emotions. These human characteristics made these divinely mysterious beings seem more rational, comprehensible, and approachable. By creating the gods in their own image, the Greeks brought into the world a more rational way of looking at love, sex, and the universe.

This mystical view created a world of fantasy, romance, and intrigue. It all seemed so attainable, and yet so mystically challenging. Therefore, the pursuit of a love, the equal of a god (soul mate), became the pursuit of nearly every man and woman throughout the ages.

It is vitally important that we be attracted to the opposite sex and that we are caught up in the whirl of romance. After all, it is the biochemical drive that keeps the world spinning! It is the electricity that draws two people together. Where and how this chemistry comes about, no one knows, but it happens! Chemistry is vitally important. Two people can meet and find each other attractive but if there isn't chemistry, nothing will happen.

The tale of Cupid and Psyche is about chemistry that knew no bounds. Cupid, the god of love and son of Venus, was willing to give up his immortal self to have the love of Psyche. Fortunately for Cupid, his father Jupiter summoned all the gods together and proclaimed, "You all know Cupid, an impetuous youth who should be curbed by some kind of bridle. He has chosen a mortal girl to be his wife. Let him keep her, and as he embraces her may he always enjoy his love."

Having said this, Jupiter ordered Psyche be brought before the gods and given a cup of nectar, the magical liquid that would make her immortal, a goddess herself. By this very act, the deep bond between Cupid and Psyche became unbreakable and eternal. Love had found its soul mate and was united eternally through the nectar of love.

The alchemists believed that the great mysteries of the soul — and love, for that matter — lay hidden under the veil of natural chemistry, and that they needed to be protected behind the physical art of alchemy. This mystical art is about removing the veil of ignorance and finding the answers to the mystery of love and life.

The love of Cupid and Psyche was made immortal through the alchemy of transferring the mortal soul into an immortal goddess. Through its test of time, the love was transmuted from an earthly presence to that of the eternal soul. In the quest for the magical elixir of life, the alchemists knew that such transformation from matter to spiritual essence was the key to the mastery of life and, thus, the mysteries of love. If it were true that behind the chemical composition of "things" lies the truth, then to find a love that transcends the mortal physical world would be to find one's soul mate.

Searching for our soul mate is much like the quest of Pygmalion, who convinced himself that women were weak, deceitful, and otherwise flawed by nature, and that no matter how hard they tried they could not overcome this curse. He was determined never to marry.

Pygmalion began working on a sculpture of a perfect young woman he called Galatea. He devoted endless hours to creating a magnificent beauty. So perfect was Galatea's creation that, against his will, he fell passionately in love with his statue. The problem he found was that although to him the statue was perfect, it was also lifeless and cold, and could not return his affections. It is as Ovid wrote; *The best art is that which conceals art.*

As luck would have it, the goddess Aphrodite turned Pygmalion's statue into a living woman, with all the characteristics of a mortal. Realizing that true beauty and love were found in the experience of life, Pygmalion married his living statue Galatea. Aphrodite blessed the nuptials she had formed, and from this union Paphos was born, from whom the city, sacred to Aphrodite, received its name.

Most mortal beings, like Psyche and Galatea, have searched for perfect and lasting love. It is the most powerful force in the universe. Nearly all of us hope to find that one person who will be our soul mate. Being in love is, of all life's experiences, the deepest. Unfortunately, many people give in to loneliness, depression, and discouragement, and settle for a person who meets only some of their needs. This usually leaves a person empty and unfulfilled.

Dr. Edward Bach, of *The Bach Flower Remedies*, declared that to have an enduring love and a passion for one's work was to have complete happiness. One without the other is only half the equation. However, if given the choice, most would choose love. When it is all said and done, very few will wish they had worked another day or made more money, but they will hope to love and make love, which is one of the deepest pleasures of being human. For in the end, all we take with us is the love we have given and the love we have received.

How do we draw love into our lives? How do we find the person who is our soul mate? It takes patience and determination. If we have taken the time to understand our own nature and the true essence of our being, then we attract the exact person for this time in our lives. If we are evolved and aware, we will be open to finding our soul mate. If we are fearful, we will draw fear and disappointment into our lives.

If the sole purpose of being is self-discovery, and self-discovery can be found only through relationships, then it would make sense that the quest to finds one's soul mate is the quest to self-discovery. However, self- discovery is a process and sometimes can take a lifetime. We can, however, hasten the process with a few natural methods such as the natural aphrodisiacs of life.

Romanticism and our culture lead us to believe that love is something we do not have and must get, so we long to experience what we see as romantic love. It is just as Galatea searched for perfection by rejecting the imperfection of the mortal world and falling in love with a perfect statue. The problem was that when he fell in love, he realized the statue was cold and lifeless and could not return his kisses and embraces.

The drive for passionate and romantic love is a universal, unconscious human need to merge with another. It is the desire, such as that found in tantra, to break down the ego and become one with another, sharing everything, including karma. It is the desire to reemerge within the universe, and, once again, become one.

However, to transcend the ego is not an easy task, for, from the ego's point of view, we are separate from the rest of the universe. We are looking out at a world that is separate from us and we must protect ourselves from it.

In yoga, it is taught that the ego is about boundaries and limitations, or *maya*, meaning illusion. Maya does not mean illusion in the sense that nothing is real. It means that our perception of reality is the illusion. We are limited only by our self-imposed boundaries, and the ego allows us to impose those boundaries. We put up walls to protect us from others, and until we learn to transcend the ego and truly connect with another, we can never find eternal love.

In relationships, we have the opportunity to become each other's mirror. We reflect exactly what we each need to learn from those closest to us. From these reflections, we have the opportunity to see both the dark and the enlightened side of ourselves. If we are brave enough to look into the reflection of relationships, we will find the true nature of our being and have the opportunity to implement change.

This is why even a so-called bad relationship is good. It provides us with the opportunity to grow, and to see both sides of ourselves. As long as we use relationships to judge others and find others' faults, rather than to discover our own strengths and weaknesses, we will be limited by the *maya*.

In the intimate and loving embrace of another, we have the opportunity to find bliss and our eternal soul. The greatest gift we can bring into a relationship is a healthy self in body, mind, and soul. By caring for our bodies and having a positive outlook, we connect again with our spiritual nature and open ourselves up to finding our soul mate. This is the ultimate chemistry of love.

In this time of contemporary relationships, the emphasis is on a strong sense of self rather than an abdication of self. When one is in union with one's own personality and spirit first, a clearer understanding of self has been established. This is the key to finding an intimate partnership that is based upon spiritual connection.

One of the greatest myths perpetuated is that of the midlife crisis and the decline of sex as we age. Psychologists such as Daniel Levinson and Erik Erikson developed models of transition in midlife. At midlife, we are confronted with the acceptance of our mortality, biological limitations, health risks, restructuring of gender identity and self-concept, reorientation to work, career, creativity and achievement, and basic life structure changes. These transitions can lead to depression, distress, and upheaval; however, there is no conclusive evidence to substantiate that midlife transition is any more of a crisis or not a crisis than any of the other transition points in our lives. Mostly it depends upon the mental outlook and the physical health of the individual.

One of the areas of transition is that of our sexual selves. Although there are physical changes at this time, the key observation is that sexual activity drops from a high of 10 or more times per month in our 20s to about three times per month at about age 65. However, a study conducted at Duke University concluded that the decline had many causes. One possibility is linked to the duration of the marriage. Studies showed that at the end of the first year of marriage sexual activity drops by half but does not drop off again for roughly another 20 years. Even though biology does play a role, such as erectile dysfunction and menopause, it also seems that decline in overall health is a major factor. Poor health, medications, and losing the mood are factors in decline.

We also experience many chemical and hormonal changes in the body. The body/brain tissue begins to decline along with the dendrites in the nerve cells. We begin to experience a loss of hearing and a decline in our vision. We find it harder to adapt to environmental changes such as stress, changes in light, and temperature variation. There is increased vulnerability to disease as the immune system works less efficiently. There is also an increased instability of biorhythms — not just the monthly cycles, but also sleep-wake patterns.

These changes are gradual, even though it seems that one day we were young and the next we hit midlife. Like all things in process, the outcome is determined by the nature of each step along the way. If we abuse our bodies in the early part of our lives, there is a pretty good chance that our midlife will show the signs. Taking care of us is a lifelong process.

Unfortunately, we don't think about these things when we are young and we feel immortal. However, since our sexual self is such an important part of enjoyment throughout our lives, it is vitally important that we support our health in natural ways. With proper nutrition, exercise, and a positive mental attitude, we can enjoy the sensual side of ourselves throughout our entire life.

Numerous studies concluded that it is not so much the lack of desire that wanes, as we get older, but rather our physical limitations due to health, as well as the lack of energy due to an unhealthy lifestyle. Rutgers University did a study on longevity and sex. They found that those who participated in regular sex, at least once a week, not only improved their physical and mental health, but also were more likely to live longer. Regular sex produces endorphins in the brain accounting for the feel-good feelings. It also causes the body to produce hormones such as human growth hormones, improving muscle tone and increasing energy. The study concluded that with regular sex we are happier, lose weight more easily, have better muscle tone, and live longer.

The Caerphilly cohort study found that 50% of those over 75 and a good percent of those younger experienced some kind of sexual difficulty. The study found that in most cases poor nutrition, poor blood circulation, and lack of essential hormones were factors. The study also concluded that mortality rate dropped by nearly 50% for those who are regularly orgasmic. The kidney function, which is also a big part of circulation, has a correlation to sexual vigor and response. The bottom line of this study is good nutrition and circulation equal a healthy appetite for sex!

There is absolutely no reason, other than a debilitating illness, that people should not be able to enjoy sex well into the latter years of life. The misconception that has been perpetuated is that sex declines as we age. Sex does not decline, it simply changes form. Throughout our lives there are many rites of passage including our sexual, sensual, physical, and psychological selves. Because this book is for adults, I am not going to write about birth, childhood, and the teenage years. I am going to start with adulthood — which we'll consider the 20s — and see if we can dispel some of the myths surrounding sex and aging.

Twenty-something. Males and females at this stage, although physically drawn to each other, are emotionally not that well suited. A woman in her 20s strives to please men so they will value her. Sexual attention becomes approval. She may look for love in all the wrong places, seeking a controlling and strong man to take the place of her parents and take care of her. This, of course, can backfire as she matures and becomes surer of herself. A

NATURALLY SEXY & HEALTHY ~ Doctor Lynn Wylnn

woman in her 20s has not reached her sexual peak. Security becomes important. The twenty-something male is at his sexual peak, and for him it is about proving himself.

While she is looking for security and romance, he is looking for sex. He believes that sex is about his success. He's detached and believes that performance, not emotional connection, is what is important. What a woman really wants at this stage is attention and intimacy. When they don't get it, they also detach, and it becomes just two warm bodies going through the motions.

Marital and relationship problems are almost inevitable at this stage. Each person is trying to find their sexuality and at the same time trying to figure out the other. Add to this the pressures of marriage, careers, and children.

Energy is high, but unfortunately, emotional understanding and the pressures of commitment can leave many couples confused and disappointed. Love and understanding can overcome many of the problems found in the twenty-something stage. The problem is, no one teaches us how to develop understanding.

Thirty-something. As young adults reach their 30s, a man's need for separateness seems to diminish. It's oftentimes just the opposite for a woman. She is now more in touch with her sexuality and perhaps a little surer of her ability to take care of herself. Often she has been married and divorced or at least been in and out of one serious relationship. It's the same for men at this age, except he may be angry, bitter, and mistrustful of women due to his feelings of rejection or failure. For a man, it is easier to find a substitute woman, even if he has no intention of a commitment. Men find it very difficult to be alone and will easily fall into a relationship without a lot of intimacy and commitment.

Then, of course, there are those who have escaped the marriage thing in their 20s. By their friends' standards, they are free and happy. However, for many unmarried people in their 30s, being unmarried may cause concern and frustration. This is a point where many people make a decision to marry because they want to stop dating or they feel this may be their last chance to marry and to have a family. These are partnerships formed mostly because of the pressure to settle down and have a family.

Forty-something. This is a stage where men and women become more compatible. Usually at this stage, they have both reached a state of sexual security and emotional maturity. She is more aggressive and orgasmic driven, he is less orgasmic driven, and more into the intimacy and touching she craved when younger. It is as if they meet at a point where the tides are shifting. The results can be more romance and better sex than ever. If a man has come to terms with his identity and a woman has learned to drop the chip from her shoulder, they can find a comfort zone that allows for a deeper level of trust and respect.

This shift has something to do with hormonal changes. As women are approaching menopause, their estrogen levels begin to drop, making testosterone stronger, which intensifies the sex drive. At the same time, the testosterone levels in a man are dropping, making him slightly less aggressive and more affectionate. Both men and women begin to experience the signs of midlife and the shift in their physical, emotional, and social priorities.

Fifty-something. If a man and woman are both healthy in this stage, they are probably for the first time equally compatible. The couple usually has more time and money combined with physical and emotional maturity. This can set the stage for great romance. However, this is also a time of great change, as both males and females go through their respective changes in life.

There are myths that as women go through menopause they cease to be interested in sex. This is not necessarily true. Depending upon a number of physical, emotional, and social factors, this can be a great time of freedom for a woman. Oftentimes it is the male who fears performance problems and backs off from the sexual encounter. If both partners understand and are caring, it can be a great time for both sexually and affectionately.

Once a man has passed through the midlife crisis, his perspective of the younger woman begins to change. Although he sees her as physically attractive, it is the wisdom and maturity of a woman his own age that holds his attraction. It is a time when for men and women, the conversation, the compatibility, and the romance is far more important than the sex. For many men in their 50s, it is the first time they find themselves turning down sex, because to them sex for the sake of sex doesn't hold its past appeal.

A woman in her 50s has developed a sense of humor and has a more carefree and secure feeling about her life. She has come to terms with her aging body and so learns to focus on other things rather than beauty and youth. She now carries a look of maturity laced with sexuality, sensuality, and wisdom. She has self-confidence, which some say is the greatest aphrodisiac of all. She makes any man of any age feel relaxed.

Sixty-something. This is a time when the fluctuation in hormones has pretty much stopped. Retirement and the pressures of family and work give way to time. If the relationship is good it only gets better, and if it is not working, it probably will end. Men become more feminine and women more masculine, bringing balance to the relationship. Although it may take a little longer for the sex to happen, when it does it is more than satisfying for both. The biggest problem regarding romance in this stage is that often women find themselves in widowhood. It can be very difficult to meet eligible men in this age group, as statistically speaking women tend to outlive men.

Beyond sixty-something. If their health is good, there is no reason why a man and a woman cannot engage in romance, love, and sex well into their 70s and 80s. Health is probably the biggest factor at this stage.

Now that we've briefly looked at the various stages of love and lust, and examined the legends and myths, let's take a look at natural aphrodisiacs.

The definition of an aphrodisiac is a substance that is used in the belief that it increases sexual desire. Throughout history, many foods, drinks, and behaviors have had a reputation for making sex more attainable and/or pleasurable. However, remember, making sex more pleasurable and attainable is not based upon taking or using one particular thing. Sexual health, and thus pleasure and desire, are based upon supporting the body-mind with a healthy lifestyle, which includes bringing vitality to your sexual self. There are many factors that contribute to sexual health.

There have been numerous substances promoted as aphrodisiacs. Some are quite farfetched, and some have grounding and validity that is based upon nutrition and other elements found in the natural world. Looking for that one silver bullet that will correct all ills is a mistake. Just like general overall health, sexual health involves balance, attitude, nutrition, exercise, herbs, color, light, sound, and scent.

Henry Kissinger said, "Power is the greatest aphrodisiac." I would say having power over your own sense of being as well as an understanding of sexual health will bring pleasure and desire into your life and may be the greatest aphrodisiac.

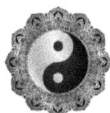

*~ A successful life: to discover a sense of adventure
in ordinary things. ~*

EROTIC FOODS

R emember our lesson in biochemistry? Nutrient-rich foodstuff and liquids are the fuel that feeds the body-mind. Our hormones, vitality, energy, thought process, state of arousal, bones, skin, blood, organs, and overall health and fitness are determined by the foods we eat and the liquids we drink. No medicine or allopathic drug supplies nutrients to the cells of our body. We need a healthy diet in order to support a healthy body-mind. Certain foods have nutritional values that support our sexual health. That is why many of these "erotic" foods have been believed to be aphrodisiacs.

Since diet is such an important part of keeping us healthy, let's take a look at some of these "erotic" foods. Keep in mind that your hormones, moods, and energy are dictated by the foods you eat, so we need to understand the role of vitamins and minerals and how we get them through the foods we eat and drink.

Vitamins and minerals are nutrients that are essential to life. They are called "micronutrients" because compared to other nutrients such as carbohydrates, fats, proteins, and water we need them in small amounts. However, it is from the foods we eat and drink that we receive these micronutrients.

Vitamins function as co-enzymes. Enzymes are the activators in the chemical reaction that break down food and allow the body to absorb and use vitamins and minerals. Without enzymes you could not breathe, walk, or make love. You need enzymes to break down proteins into essential amino acids and for nerve transmission. For example, a particular enzyme needs B6 vitamin to activate it, so this enzyme and vitamin can transmit nerve impulses to your fingers. If you are deficient in B6, the transmission of your nerve impulses may be weak causing numbness in your fingers.

Minerals are also needed to activate proper composition of body fluids, blood, and bone formation, and to maintain a healthy nervous system. Where do these vitamins and minerals come from? The foods we eat. So doesn't it make sense that our sexual health involves a sexy healthy diet?

Toxic chemicals in the environment have been a suspect in male infertility. Sperm counts in the United States have declined by as much as 80 percent over the last fifty years. However, vitamin C has been shown to increase the percentage of normal sperm, sperm mortality, and sperm vitality in fertile men with lower sperm count.

Again, it is fair to say that a healthy diet is needed to ensure a healthy sex life. Diet alone will not make you a master lover but without a healthy diet, we can see that the body-mind is missing important nutrients that support sexual health. If you really want to find aphrodisiacs, you need look no further than your kitchen cupboard. Nature has endowed us with many foods that enhance and support sexual health.

Histamine, a neurotransmitter that increases arousal, is responsible for the flush of blood that rushes to the surface of the skin when we are aroused. Researchers have found that foods containing B5 vitamin (pantothenic acid, the anti-stress vitamin) and rutin can actually raise histamine levels. B5 vitamin is found in liver, peanuts, mushrooms, peas, eggs, oatmeal, brewer's yeast, sunflower seeds, lentils, brown rice, whole wheat, fresh vegetables, and salmon. Foods supplying rutin include broccoli, grapes, all citrus and tropical fruits, cherries, cabbage, parsley, melon, and peppers.

Niacin (B3) is another erotic vitamin. It enhances sexual pleasure for both males and females. It causes the blood vessels closest to the skin to widen and fill with blood. The result is a warm tingling feeling that extends from the neck and the ears to the torso and on down to the genital region. The niacin-induced effect makes the skin feel more alive and more sensitive to touch, which helps to heighten the physical sensations of lovemaking. This erotic vitamin helps oxytocin to do its job by heightening the sensation of touch. Niacin is found in sesame seeds, peanuts, lean beef, barley, split peas, shrimp, haddock, eggs, broccoli, peaches, tomatoes, and carrots.

Inadequate nutrition seems to have a direct link to hormone production. One of the tasks of the sex hormones is to stimulate vaginal lubrication and penile erection. One of the ways to increase this is with vitamin B6, which is involved in the production of estrogen and testosterone. B6 aids in maintaining potassium and sodium levels and producing serotonin. It is required by the nervous system, and is needed for normal brain function, and for the synthesis of RNA and DNA, which contain the genetic instruction for the reproduction and growth of normal cells. Foods rich in B6 are lima beans and kidney beans, chicken, fish, eggs, spinach, peas, avocado, tuna, hazelnuts, bananas, Brussels sprouts, sweet potatoes, and cauliflower. Antidepressants, estrogen, and oral contraceptives may increase the need for B6.

There is increasing evidence that perimenopause symptoms can be treated nutritionally. Studies show that the loss of sex drive a woman experiences may be due to nutritional deficiencies caused by the body stress of the sudden loss of estrogen. A poor diet affects our weight, our moods, and our energy levels. It should be stated that a good nutritional diet is not only essential to our health, but is essential to our sexual health. Studies have shown that adding soy products such as tofu and sage, vitamin E, ginseng, calcium, zinc, vitamin C, and the B-complex vitamins — promises to be an excellent way to naturally treat the symptoms of menopause by raising estrogen levels.

Vegetables (leafy greens), legumes (soybeans), and ginseng contain phytoestrogens that can be very beneficial. When estrogen levels are low in the body, phytoestrogens are able to exert some estrogenic activity, and when estrogen levels are high, phytoestrogens reduce overall estrogen activity by occupying estrogen receptor sites. This may explain why Asian women seem to experience less severe menopausal symptoms. It is vitally important to remember that we can sabotage our energy levels by eating processed foods, sugars, and drinking alcohol and caffeine. All of these have the potential to lower energy, and cause depression.

Calcium is another important supplement but should be taken with magnesium. Calcium and magnesium together ensure the uptake of these important minerals. Not only does calcium help build strong bones and teeth, it also activates the enzyme that helps us digest fat and protein and assists in the production of energy. Foods rich in calcium are dairy, sardines, salmon, and leafy greens.

Vitamin E is extremely important to both sexes as an antioxidant. It seems that vitamin E deficiencies found in animals show signs of testicular degeneration and sterility. Vitamin E has also been shown to be helpful in reducing hot flashes and improving PMS symptoms. Hot flashes, are caused by the sudden withdrawal of estrogen.

It is interesting to note than many of the foods that are phytoestrogens also are rich in vitamin E. Good food sources are natural vegetable oils, legumes, soybeans, dark leafy vegetables, grains, brown rice, salmon, and eggs. Perhaps this is why vitamin E has been reputed to be the "sex vitamin."

Two erotic minerals that may enhance your sex life are zinc and selenium. Oysters, reputed to be an aphrodisiac, are rich in zinc and selenium. Men especially need to get adequate zinc. Each time a man ejaculates, he loses about 1 milligram of zinc through the sperm. Zinc-rich foods are shellfish, milk, oats, green beans, yams, cucumbers, lentils, garlic, potatoes, fish, tuna, black beans, nuts, liver, eggs, and anchovies. Selenium is found in mushrooms, onions, kidney beans, peas, grapes, most shellfish, organ meats, meats, wheat germ, bran, and cottage cheese.

For most of us, we depend upon the richness of the soil to get these important minerals. Plants draw minerals from the soil and pass then up the food chain. If the soil is deficient in zinc and selenium, the plants, and thus the food chain, will be deficient. As supplements incorporated into our diets, these two minerals increase the stimulation response, libido, and sexual arousal in both men and women.

There is one part of the brain that is essential for taking care of fatty products in the system: the so-called sex brain. The sex drive is located in the limbic system, which, along with the rest of the brain, depends upon 400 calories per day in the right proportion of nutrients for proper functioning. If we starve the sex brain of needed nutrients, it can't direct the body into proper performance. The brain and nerves need a certain substance called neurolin. When the sex brain is weak, neurolin cannot be assimilated or utilized. This substance supports memory, the utilization of fat, and initiating the faculty of affection. Potassium is needed to ensure that this substance is secreted. It is vitally important to our health and our sexual selves to keep the pH (acid-alkaline) levels of our blood in balance. Potassium and sodium help us to achieve this state. Your body, optimally, should be slightly more alkaline than acid. It is reputed that a mixture of oats and raw egg yolk, which has iron and phosphorous, along with sleep, will cure impotence in men and women. An oatmeal diet, which also helps to keep away depression and lift moods, is recommended for retaining an affectionate state. Herbalists actually use the oat plant to treat depression. Oatmeal brings the body back to an alkaline state, which is good for nerve transmission, and thus, our sexual health.

Chocolate has been found to contain constituents that enhance affection, elevate our mood, and give us that "in love" sensation. The reason for this is that chocolate contains a substance known as phenylethylamine or PEA. It's our old friend, PEA, that brings on the amphetamine-like rush of chemistry. Because this fattening aphrodisiac is known to flood our brain with sexual excitement, in ancient times it was forbidden to nuns, but consumed without restraint by priests.

Although chocolate is sweet, and it does contain the "love" peptide, it doesn't remain in our system for long, if it is fat and sugar-laden like most candy. When we refer to chocolate as an aphrodisiac, we're talking about the dark rich pure chocolate of the cocoa plant.

Avocados are storehouses of nutrients. They are full of potassium, sulfur, phosphorous, and magnesium. The avocado supplies energy and sexual desire. Why? Because it is loaded with, the minerals and vitamins needed to support a healthy sexual system.

Watercress, frequently found on plates because of its bright green color, is a wonderful source of vitamins and minerals. It is full of iron, magnesium, calcium, phosphorous, sulfur, vitamins A, B1, B2, C, and the mineral zinc.

Actually, you need look no further than your spice rack to find a host of nature's aphrodisiacs. Spices are more than simply condiments for your foods. If we talk about spicing up our lives, cloves, cinnamon, sage, black pepper, and nutmeg are a few of the erotic spices sitting quietly in your cupboard just waiting for your indulgence. The following "sex tonic" is said to spice up your life. It is not too far-fetched when you consider that celery is an alkaline food known for its sodium content, which is what we call the "youth maintainer" of our body.

CELERY TONIC

- Put four pieces of celery in a pot of boiling water Steep for twenty minutes
- Add chopped clove of garlic
- Sprinkle black pepper, nutmeg, and cinnamon on top
- Add a heaping teaspoon of honey
- Stir and drink a shot every three hours.

Or, take the yellowish oil that is extracted from the celery root and mix three drops with a teaspoon of honey and drink twice daily. Black pepper, nutmeg, and cinnamon are sexual-energy–enhancing spices. Their warm and stimulating properties help to pump blood to sexual organs.

Growing up, you were probably told to eat your fruits and vegetables because they would make you strong. It is doubtful that your parents were referring to your ability in the bedroom; however, vegetables and fruits do improve our virility. Perhaps you have heard of the doctrine of signatures. It means that foods take on a look similar to the properties they enhance. For example, asparagus, bananas, and figs all have a phallic look. But as well as looking sexy, they also supply sexy nutrients. Bananas, with their potassium content, help to keep the muscular system strong. They also contain phosphorous, protein, niacin, and fat, all good for the sexual system. Figs, the so-called "female fruit," are high in a natural sugar that creates energy. They are also a high-calcium food.

All we need to do is look at the shape of the asparagus, with its long erect body, to appreciate its erotic properties. It contains asparagine, which imparts a strong odor in the urine. Steam your asparagus and save the water. Drink about two ounces each evening before going to bed for one week. It is said this will improve your virility. Try boiling artichokes until the leaves can be easily removed. Then boil goat's milk for three minutes. Sprinkle some nutmeg on top and add a little honey and then eat the leaves. Supposedly, this recipe will instill lust in even the most tranquil people. High in calcium, iron, vitamins A and C, and niacin, it is easy to see why this is a sensual food.

Shiitake mushrooms contain D3, which closely resembles certain hormones that may account for their effect on sexual excitement. For men, erectile dysfunction is an inability of the blood to engorge the tissue in the penis sufficiently to ensure erection. This comes with aging, disease, and stress. According to folklore, shiitakes can correct this situation. Shiitakes also have a stimulating effect on females by making the nipples redder and more responsive.

A fleshy edible underground fungus known as truffles has erotic abilities that date back to the time of the Romans. The early Romans traded gold and jewels for Libyan truffles because of their powerful action and more pleasant taste. In ancient times, truffles were fed to both men and women as an aphrodisiac.

The ancient Romans also swore by the erectile ability of arugula. Arugula is a good source of iron and calcium. It has a bittersweet taste that can turn any salad into an erotic experience.

Strawberries, long known as the fruit of lovers, are high in fiber and vitamin C. They are an excellent spring tonic, meaning they help to tone and strengthen the system. Because of their high sodium content, they are considered "a food for youth," building strength and virility. Strawberries are chockfull of erotic vitamins and minerals.

Onions and garlic are high in sulfur. Because of its ability to protect against the harmful effects of radiation and pollution, sulfur can slow down the aging process. Sulfur is found in the hemoglobin and all body tissue, and is needed for the synthesis of collagen, which prevents dryness and maintains elastins in the skin. Take one teaspoon of onion juice three or four times a day or soak half an onion in a cup of water for two days. Strain and drink half a cup daily. Garlic, onions, aloe, leeks, and watercress are a few of the high-sulfur foods.

Did you know that wild lettuce contains lactucarium, an alkaloid drug? When allowed to go to seed, lettuce contains a milky juice that has a mild narcotic effect and promotes feelings of sexual stimulation.

Eat your oat bran! Oats are a stimulant, nerve cell nutrient, and nerve tonic. In China, oats are given as an agent for impotency due to overindulgence in sex. It is said that they produce a tonic effect on the nerves of the sensual organs. Oats are excellent tonics used to treat depression and nervous disorders. They are also known for their strength-building properties. Try 15 drops of oat fluid extract in a glass of water three times a day.

Caviar and fish eggs are exceptional aphrodisiacs. What we do know about fish is that it is high in the erotic mineral zinc. Caviar is also high in phosphorous, which transforms into metabolic activity and penile erections.

However, phosphorous obtained from the earth is poisonous to us. It must be transformed through another organism, and this is just what the sturgeons do for us.

Many foods add health to our sexual life but one food has been used throughout history as a sexual stimulant and energy provider. Honey — the nectar of the bees!

Honey has all it takes to improve your sex life. Honey, when used appropriately or combined with other food items, promotes growth and regeneration of body tissues and strengthen a healthy physical body. It is therefore not an overstatement that honey can miraculously improve your sex life in many ways.

Pure and unheated honey is a mild sexual stimulant since it contains numerous substances such as vitamin E, B6, thiamin, niacin, riboflavin, pantothenic acid, and certain amino acids. The minerals found in honey include calcium, copper, iron, magnesium, manganese, phosphorus, potassium, sodium, and zinc, which promote virility and reproductive health. In England, mead, which is made from honey, was considered an aphrodisiac. It was drunk for a month before the wedding, to make the couple sexually potent. This is the origin of the word *honeymoon.*

Whether it be sexual, athletic, or everyday energy output, performance is important. Having strength, endurance, and quick recovery time, as well as an enhanced state of mind, is conducive to winning any of the games of life or, for that matter, the sexual dance. You can perfect your skills and have tremendous talent, but if you do not give your body and mind the nutrients it needs, your performance will fail.

In 1955, research done by the Sports College of Canada found that one food supplied the energy and nutrients needed to both sustain performance and bring about quick recovery. When tested against other energy foods, it ranked number one. In ranking the foods, the researchers took into consideration:

1. measurable reaction
2. digestibility
3. chemical reaction (acidity, etc.)
4. general tolerance of athlete to food concerned
5. caloric content per serving
6. taste appeal
7. versatility
8. economy
9. basic ingredients.

This complete food was ideal: it was versatile, as it could be combined with many products; was easily digestible; and apparently was free of bacteria and irritating substances. The vitamin content in this food included B1, B2, C (ascorbic acid), and pantothenic acid. All of these vitamins and minerals acted as antioxidants, protecting the body from free radical formation. This food, of course, was honey, the nectar of the gods!

If we take a practical look at our health, it is easy to see that good nutrition is essential to living a long, radiant, vital, and vigorous life. Food in its natural form is the foundation of health. Fast food, processed foods, and overeating are major problems in today's world. Obesity and ill health have a direct connection to poor diet. Our sexual health depends upon good nutrition.

Food or foodstuff also includes herbs and spices. Let us look now at the world of sexual herbs and spices.

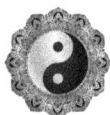

*~ A successful life: to teach, to share,
to give without looking for a return. ~*

HERBS, SPICES, AND OILS

In earlier times, herbs and spices were considered luxuries and only available for use by the wealthy. In medieval times, herbs and spices were also traded frequently between tribes and countries. Many people do not know the difference between an herb and a spice. The debate between herbs and spices is ongoing. Some say that there is no difference, while others maintain that they are completely different.

The essential difference is where it is obtained on a plant. Herbs usually come from the leafy part of a plant, and are usually dried. However, some herbs can be used fresh. Spices are typically from seeds, fruits, roots, bark, or some other vegetative substance. Herbs can be found many places around the world, while spices are more commonly found in the Far East and tropical countries. Herbs are considered to have more uses than spices.

For instance, herbs have been used medicinally more frequently than spices. Also, herbs can and have been used to augment cosmetics and preserve foods.

Because herbs and spices have so many uses and are great food flavorings, they have played important roles throughout history. The Portuguese navigator, Vasco Da Gama, sailed to India in search of spices. Even Christopher Columbus described the types of spices available in the "new world." Herbs have been used throughout history for medicinal purposes. In traditional Chinese medicine, herbology has been used for thousands of years.

Throughout history, herbs and spices have also played a major part in the making of aphrodisiacs. If we look closely at herbs and spices, and keep in mind that they are plants and, thus, foodstuff made up of proteins, carbohydrates, fats, sugars and essential vitamins and minerals, their use as aphrodisiacs has a ring of truth.

Marjoram, myrtle, acacia, cyprus, and garcinia are herbs that are also used in potions or by themselves as aphrodisiacs. Their roots can be boiled in a stew and their precious oils used for massages.

Along with the licorice root, the Chinese use schizandra berries and lycii berries as aphrodisiacs. Both berries are vibrant red in color and a bit sour. Steep them in hot water and add licorice root to sweeten.

Three of history's most famous lovers are Don Juan, Casanova, and Cleopatra. Each purported to have had secret love potions, which made it impossible for their lovers to resist their affections.

According to written reports, Don Juan was said to mix and drink the following passion potion to restore his potency after hours of lustful lovemaking. He mixed it fresh and took it one hour before his next encounter.

Take 1/4 teaspoon of crushed fresh basil leaves and one cup of freshly squeezed tomato juice. Mix furiously so that the basil oil is released into the drink. Sip slowly.

We cannot be sure that this was the entire potion; however, basil is an herb that builds strength in the physical body and is used for alleviating mental fatigue. Fresh tomato juice is rich in sodium (a strength-builder), calcium, potassium, and magnesium. The citric, malic, and oxalic acid found in tomato juice is good for metabolism.

Casanova, another infamous lover, was said to have kept a mysterious royal purple vase beside his bed, containing a mysterious liquid. To his guest he offered wine, but for himself he only drank from the mysterious vase.

After his death, it is said that a young chemist stole the vase and discovered the mysterious elixir of love. What he found was grapefruit juice, steamed apple juice, and cinnamon powder mixed vigorously. Again, perhaps this was not the entire elixir, but we do know that apples are an alkaline food, good for elimination, circulation, and helping the body to absorb and effectively use iron. Grapefruit juice, another alkaline fruit, is also good for circulation and aids digestion. The Chinese, to promote circulation and internal energy, have long used cinnamon. It is said to increase *yang* energy and thus sexual vitality. The three ingredients together help to promote good digestion and circulation, which are essential to feeling strong and healthy, and this in turn is essential to a vibrant sexual self.

First, there was the fall of Julius Caesar, and then Marc Anthony. Legend has it that Cleopatra used potions to lure and seduce her men. When she sailed to meet Marc Anthony, she soaked the sails of her ship in jasmine oil, one of the most intense aphrodisiac fragrances. Marc Anthony fell so deeply in love with Cleopatra that he gave up his kingdom for her.

Supposedly, Cleopatra would go on 24-hour fasts where she would take nothing but her elixir of love, reemerging from her boudoir to give and receive another 24 hours of pleasure.

The following recipe has been called Cleopatra's secret love formula. It tastes great and is a great refreshing drink.

Blend 1/2 cup of frozen banana, a couple of small ice cubes, 1/4 cup seedless watermelon, 1/2 cup ripened papaya chunks, 1/2 teaspoon each, powdered cloves and cinnamon, 1/4 cup of kefir or non-fat plain yogurt and 1/8 cup orange juice at a high speed until thoroughly mixed. Sip slowly.

This mixture is not too far-fetched, as careful examination of its contents reveals a mixture of fruits high in vitamins and minerals and antioxidants that support and stimulate the sex glands and hormones.

Humans have sought aphrodisiacs since the beginning of time. Claims of allure, lust, and love have been attributed to many elixirs and magical potions. If you read carefully the science behind our sexual nutrition, you will see that many of these potions are not too far off from reality. This all goes to prove that a healthy diet and exercise are probably the greatest aphrodisiacs of all! The world of herbs and spices invites sensual delight and pleasure. Herbs and spices, we must remember, are simply "foodstuff." They are comprised of the same essential nutrients as fruits and vegetables, such as essential vitamins and minerals, proteins, carbohydrates, fats, and sugars. There is a reason why herbs and spices have been used to season and enhance foods; they enhance your sexual health! However, if you are taking MAO inhibitors or certain medicines prescribed for high blood pressure and cardiac disease, some herbs may be harmful. Always check with your primary physician before mixing herbs and drugs.

Here are a few of my favorite lustful herbs.

Sage is an herb that is reputed to guarantee long life and is known to mimic female hormones. Sage can be used daily; 1–2 cups per day of tea as a natural supplement. St. John's wort can be used daily as an antidepressant, along with vervain. Dill seed herb is frequently used with other herbs in love potions. Steep a little in a cup of hot water for a sensual drink. It is a great herb for digestive problems and acts as a calmative.

Pure vanilla from the vanilla bean has a wonderful aroma that has an aphrodisiac effect. Steep a vanilla pod in a good brandy for three weeks and then have a shot. It is sure to relax and stimulate.

One herb that has been used as an aphrodisiac and has gotten a lot of attention is **yohimbie**, a substance derived from the bark of an African evergreen tree. Yohimbie was tested at Stanford University and Queen's University where it was given the label as a true aphrodisiac. The problem with yohimbie is that when it is combined with any allopathic drugs, it has the potential to do harm. The Food and Drug Administration does not consider it to be an aphrodisiac and does not feel it is safe to use so it is difficult to find. The FDA prohibits marketing any over-the-counter product that claims it "Improves sex life, helps restore sexual vigor, and builds virility and sexual potency." However, over-the-counter supplements that enhance health are okay to market. So does that make it okay to market sexual health supplements? Confusing as it may be, Viagra with no nutritional content and adverse side effects is given with approval by the FDA!

Ginseng is another herb that is highly valued as a treatment for impotency. Ginseng is known for its ability to restore virility and strength. It does not appear to stimulate the sex glands into unnatural activity. It is used as a restorer of sexual function that has become tired and weary. Ginseng is used for lack of virility and energy, fatigue, and mental and physical exhaustion. Now I ask you, don't all of the above (exhaustion, fatigue, etc.) affect your sex life?

Ginseng's remedial effects on sex are not immediate. In fact, the Chinese maintain that the herb is not to be classified as an aphrodisiac because it does not immediately stimulate activity. Ginseng rebuilds and restores healthy functioning. The chemical and nutrient content of ginseng is calcium, camphor, ginosides, iron, resin, starch, and vitamins A, B12, and E. Aren't these all nutrients that increase performance and improve vitality, mood, ability to concentrate, and improve motor control? Doesn't it seem that improved overall performance might be helpful in the bedroom?

The Chinese frequently prescribe **licorice root** as a marital aid. Among its many nutritional contents are biotin, fat, manganese, PABA, pantothenic acid, phosphorus, protein, sugar, and vitamins B1, B2, B3, B4, B5, B6, B9, and E. It also has estrogenic substances that may account for its sexual stimulation properties.

Sarsaparilla is not to be confused with the soda sasparille, a popular drink in the Old West during the 1820–1890s. Sarsaparilla is a medicinal herb used to treat such complaints as arthritis, herpes, psoriasis, eczema, leprosy, and syphilis. No peer groups have reviewed these claims. There is peer research suggesting that it has antioxidant properties. Sarsaparilla's nutrient contents are copper, fat, iron, manganese, resin, saponins, sodium, sugar, sulfur, vitamins A and D, and zinc. Do you remember these nutrients from the chapter on erotic foods? These nutrients give you energy, strength, and vitality. When I was young, I remember having sasparille soda. There was something sweetly erotic about it. It tasted somewhat like vanilla. That is why people love sarsaparilla.

Hops, the herb used in the beer-brewing process, is not known for its ability to enhance lovemaking. The hop plant, however, is a close relative of the cannabis (marijuana) plant. If smoked like a joint it will produce a mild high accompanied by a sense of serenity. Although the hop is calming, its lupulin substance, a close relative to THC (marijuana), accounts for its ability to present everything in a better light and let the libido say "hello, baby." However, remember, herbs can be dangerous, so it is always best to seek medical advice, and remember more is not necessarily better. Among its nutrients, a hop contains asparagines, manganese, PABA, resin, and vitamin B6. B6 is needed for healthy blood. A deficiency has been linked to depression and lack of energy. Healthy blood levels, a happy mood, and energy are all essential for a healthy sex life.

Oat straw is another medicinal herb. It is considered a valuable remedy for strengthening and restoring nerve energy. In China, oats are given as an agent for impotency due to overindulgence in sex. Oat straw is used to treat depression and nervous disorders. Some studies indicate that oats are a male stimulant. According to James Duke, Ph.D., when wild stallions eat oats they supposedly become friskier and libidinous, which is where we get the phrase "sowing wild oats." There is also the definition of "sowing your wild oats" that means to idle away time by separating the useful and unuseful parts of the oat plant.

Schizandra is considered a powerful sexual tonic. It is also believed that schizandra berries have strong liver-supporting properties.

Now my favorite of all erotic herbs is **damiana** (pronounced dame-me- anna). Used for weakness, exhaustion, and nervousness, it also has been used for increasing the sperm count in men and strengthening the ovaries in women. Damiana is an herb used as a sexual stimulant, circulation booster, diuretic, and muscle relaxant. Modern chemistry has identified a number of chemical constituents such as alkaloid damiana, which stimulates nerves and sexual organs. It also contains arbutin, resin, starch, sugar, and tannins.

The ancient Aztecs used the herb as a tonic and a cure for impotence. The leaves are smooth and pale green. The flowers are yellow and have an aromatic smell with a bitter taste. Somewhat like good sex — smooth and aromatic with a bite.

One last herb to consider, although there are numerous herbs we could add to this list: marijuana has long been considered an aphrodisiac. Ayurvedic medicine (an ancient Indian medicine, the oldest still-existing practice) used **cannabis** to increase libido, produce long-lasting erections, delay ejaculation, facilitate lubrication, and loosen inhibitions. Morocco, Egypt, Lebanon, and other Middle Eastern and North African cultures used cannabis for sexual purposes in a potent form known as *Kif* as recently as the 20th century.

Cannabis heightens the senses, relaxes you, and makes you feel hyper connected. Brain chemistry, hormones, and the sex regions of the brain are affected by marijuana. That is because THC (delta 9-Tetrahydrocannabinol), the active ingredient in marijuana, releases dopamine in the brain, causing a high, and replicates a sexy little neurochemical called anandamide. However, for some people marijuana makes them introspective and contemplative, which is the opposite effect. They would rather meditate than copulate! But this varies from person to person. Heavy long-term use does appear to diminish sex drive as well as motivation. With all things, moderation is best.

It is true that the cells of the reproductive system are high in fat, and this absorbs more THC than other cells. However, there have been no epidemiological studies to indicate that reproductive rates are any higher or lower in countries where high usage of marijuana is found. Like everything in life, moderation is the key. I live in California where medical marijuana is legal. It is used medicinally for depression, anxiety, cancer, AIDS, IBS, glaucoma, pain, and other digestive, painful, and restless disorders. Perhaps with a little more study, it will be used for sexual disorders so that the side effects of Viagra and other sexual enhancers can be avoided and a natural approach can be taken.

Now let us jump past the herbs and into a few spices. There is a reason beyond taste as to why spices were added to foods and drinks. Yes, they made things smell better, taste better, and they helped to preserve, but they also tantalized the libido. Now remember, the essential difference between an herb and a spice is where they are found on the plant. Herbs usually come from the leafy part of a plant, and are usually dried. However, some herbs can be used fresh. Spices can be obtained from seeds, fruits, roots, bark, or some other vegetative substance.

There is an erotic shop just waiting inside your spice cupboard. Open the door and take a whiff. Throughout history, spices have been used to enhance and delight. Here are a few of the so-called "sex" spices.

Cinnamon has long been used by the Chinese as a powerful tonic spice. It's warm and stimulating properties improve circulation and regulate blood sugar levels. Research conducted at the Smell & Taste Treatment & Research Foundation in Chicago concluded that when men smelled foods such as pumpkin pie and cinnamon buns (foods with the most cinnamon), blood flow increased, suggesting cinnamon could help with penile erections. New studies also show that cinnamon speeds up the brain's processing of visual cues. We all know that men are more visual than women, so if you want to please your man, bake him a pumpkin pie, cinnamon buns, or sprinkle cinnamon on his oatmeal in the morning. The sight of the cinnamon bun or pie will excite him and the smell will captivate him.

Cloves are also a strong spice for circulation. Like cinnamon, cloves are warming and stimulating. Bake a ham stuffed with cloves for a sensual dinner.

Coriander seeds are stimulants. This spice is often added to Moroccan food. Pepper is also a stimulating spice. Peppers have oils that stimulate the heat- sensing nerves of the skin and mucous membranes. When these oils arrive at the sex sites (genitourinary), they create heat and stimulate sensations.

Saffron is a wonderfully aromatic spice that could also be an herb. It is noted for its aphrodisiac ability. It takes 225,000 handpicked stigmas from the saffron crocus to make a single pound, making saffron the world's most expensive spice. Saffron-based pigments dating back 5,000 years have been found in modern-day Iraq. Iranians, or Persians, used the spice medicinally as well as to treat melancholy and to stimulate the libido. It is said that non- Persians feared the Persians' use of saffron as an aphrodisiac. Saffron is comprised of 150 aromatic oils and other aromatic substances. Its yellow color is the result of a-crocin. A-crocin is a carotenoid that breaks down into other carotenoids, one of which is zeaxanthin, which happens to be one of the carotenoids found in the retina of the human eye. Carotenoids are red, yellow, and orange fat-soluble pigments found in many plants that are powerful antioxidants and related to vitamin A. Now, we know vitamin A supports the immune system. It's also responsible for the formation of epithelial tissue, which is found almost everywhere on the body including the skin, glands, mucous membranes, the lining of the hollow organs, and along the entire respiratory, gastrointestinal, and genitourinary tracts. Need I say more about saffron?

The Arab world considered **cardamom** a stimulating spice. It contains at least two androgenic (male) compounds. Cardamom is a great source of cineole, a compound that stimulates the nervous system. Drop a dash into your coffee or tea for a tasty stimulating drink.

Nutmeg is a spice that is found in most kitchens, known for its distinct aroma and flavor. It is prepared from the ground seed of the tropical evergreen plant. Mace, another spice, is made from the outer covering of the nutmeg. The Dutch introduced the nutmeg seeds to the Europeans in the early part of the 17th century. The people who settled America brought the spice with them and it has become common in American cuisine. However, it also has a sinister side because not only does it enhance food, it's also a sedative, a mind-altering substance, and an aphrodisiac. Most herbs and spices in large doses can be poisonous and mind-altering. Nutmeg is no exception. The substances, which make it more than a spice, are elemicin, myristicin, and safrole. A little bit sprinkled on your pudding can entice a spicy romp in the hay, but a large dose can make you very sick. Just a little dash will do to create a sexy and sensual dessert.

What other spices and herbs are sitting on your shelf awaiting a taste-filled, sexy meal? They are curry, basil, ginger, parsley, fennel, fenugreek, and a lot more!

Herbs and spices are a wonderful way to tantalize the taste buds and excite the olfactory nerves. Taste and smell are essential elements in the dance of lust and love. However, when it comes to smells the use of essential oils or aromatherapy has the power to subtly affect our lustful self. Essential oils of all kinds have been used ritualistically since the dawn of time. Some anthropologists believe that the birth of human culture began with some form of ritual using herbs, spices, and oils to scent the air. These aromatic herbs, flowers, and spices were used to fumigate, as antiseptics, and to act on a more subtle level for psychic and spiritual healing. Modern aromatherapy was born in France at the turn of the 20th century. Essential oils were studied for their medicinal properties. Essential oils have hundreds of chemical compounds, most in very small amounts. Like the herbs, plants, flowers, and trees that these essential oils come from, nature has bestowed proteins, sugars, nutrients, and healing compounds within the essence of the oils. There are many well-known documented uses of essential oils being used medicinally to treat a host of maladies, mostly for fumigation and as antiseptics.

Since this is a book about sex, we will just focus on the so-called aphrodisiac oils. However, two things need to be understood. Essential oils are extractions of what is considered the lifeblood of the plant. The oils are the essence or purest form of plant energy. The oils are very concentrated and should be used carefully. Never use them directly on the skin or take them internally. If you wish to use essential oils medicinally, seek out a qualified practitioner.

Second, we must get a brief lesson in how the olfactory system works. Our sense of smell acts mostly on a subconscious level. The olfactory nerves are directly connected to our primitive brain, or the limbic system. Our limbic system, originally known as the rhinencephalon system (smell brain), is the part of the brain that regulates sensory motor activity and deals with the primitive drives of sex, hunger, and thirst. Stimulation of the olfactory nerves through the sense of smell sends electrical signals to the limbic system, directly affecting sex, digestion, and emotional behavior. Think about when you walk into a mall and smell cinnamon buns. It makes you think of eating. On the other hand, the smell of flowers gives us a subtle mental lift. Now, think how you react to something that smells foul? All animals release sexual olfactory signals called pheromones.

Remember our old friend DHEA? It's what gives us our unique smell. When we are born, it is the sense of smell that attaches us to our mothers. Our hormones also influence our sense of smell and the way we smell to others. Do you remember from earlier in this book that women have a better sense of smell than men do? That is because the hormone estrogen enhances our sense of smell.

Fragrances are molecules that emit a scent from just about everything. These fragrances have their own language. Better than any words, the scent expresses the most subtle sensations and feelings. Try to express in words the smell of wild lavender or a beautiful rose. How about chocolate? What does chocolate smell like? There are no words, to accurately express, what a scent smells like.

During the Renaissance, the *grande dames* had their own secret perfumes. Cleopatra used jasmine and other scents to seduce her lovers. Essential oils used medicinally enhance sensuality by subtly stimulating the olfactory with subconscious fragrant messages. However, like all natural therapies, essential oils do not work in isolation. Combined with all the other natural therapies, like diet and exercise, an organism establishes balance and thus health.

Let us look at some of the sensuality-enhancing essential oils. First here is how it works. Essential oils are extracted from plants and then mixed with oils, creams, waxes, or sometimes used directly without any additives. Remember oils, like herbs, come from plants and as such are living organisms. They have chemical compounds such as phenols, esters, and aldehydes as well as proteins, sugars, and fats. Now, we do not want to get bogged down with all the science behind essential oils, but it is important tonote that oils have antiseptic, astringent, and soothing properties. If you would like to learn more about essential oils and aromatherapy, go to www.colourenergy.com or DoTerra Essential Oils (www.doterraoil.com).

The main aphrodisiac oils are jasmine, ylang ylang, pepper, sandalwood, patchouli, cardamom, cloves, clary sage, nutmeg, and musk.

The olfactory nerves (inside the nasal passage) connect with the limbic part of the brain. In fact, the olfactory passageway is the most direct pathway to the brain. We breathe in an odor and immediately it registers in the brain. Certain scents are said to stimulate the sex center. Mammals, remember, release sexual olfactory signals called pheromones through special scent- producing apocrine glands. In humans, most of these glands are located in the abdomen and chest area, most notably around the nipples.

Scents that mimic the olfactory signals are musk, sandalwood, and civet. Therefore, the main function of perfumes should be to heighten and fortify the natural sexual scents rather than to mask them. But since the human pheromones are nearly undetectable, aromatic sensual scents have been employed to attract lovers. The connection between olfaction and sexual systems takes place through the hypothalamic region of the brain.

The hypothalamic region is a major receiver of olfactory neurons; it releases a variety of hormones, which pass to the anterior pituitary via the hypophyseal portal system, and induces the pituitary to secrete the suite of hormones, which governs and controls the mammalian sexual cycles. Wow!

And now the oils...

My favorite sexual essential oil is **ylang ylang,** which is sweet, voluptuous, and exotic. It means flower of flower. In Indonesia, people spread ylang ylang flowers on the bed of newly married couples on their wedding night.

Pepper, one of the most ancient spices, is strong, hot, and vital. It has a strong scent, which is good for impotence, strength, and fortitude.

Jasmine is another oil to which I am absolutely addicted. Whenever I am drawn to a commercial perfume, it usually contains jasmine, ylang ylang, vanilla, or a combination. Jasmine is deep, warm, exhilarating, and exotic. Sensually speaking, jasmine might be the best aphrodisiac aromatherapy can offer. Jasmine is said to release inhibitions, liberate imaginations, and develop exhilarating playfulness. It is also believed that the power of jasmine can be experienced only by true lovers, as it has the power to transcend physical love and fully release both male and female sexual energy.

Nutmeg, cloves, cardamom, and cinnamon have warming and stimulating properties. Just like their spice properties, the scent of these warming essential oils aids digestion and stimulates sexual desires. Medicinally they have been used for impotence and circulation.

Patchouli is a product of India, Malaysia, Burma, and Paraguay. When you think of patchouli, you may think of it as a perfume used by Indians to treat their fabrics or as an incense used to disguise the smell of cannabis that floated around your dorm room. It is a warm plant used medicinally by the Chinese and the Indians as a tonic for digestive issues and as a stimulant for sluggishness and inertia. The smell of patchouli in the air moves through the olfactory and into the limbic system where it stimulates the nervous system positively. It sets the mood for sex.

Sandalwood is another "hippie" scent. Sandalwood is mentioned in the ancient Sanskrit and Chinese books. It was used widely in religious ceremonies. Its woody, spicy, sweet scent is supposedly good for impotence. Sandalwood and musky scents, according to D.M. Stoddard, contain an ingredient similar to androstenol, a male pheromone.

Clary sage, produced in Southern France, is used primarily by women to alleviate frigidity. It is a phytoestrogen, meaning it has estrogenic properties. That is why it is a good sexual oil for women.

There are many more scents that we could discuss, but this covers the top sexual and sensual oils. When purchasing perfumes, gravitate to the scent and then look at the blend of oils that make up the aroma. You may be surprised by the choice you make.

In the spiritual approach to aromatherapy, essential oils are considered the life force or the energy of the plant. Alchemists regarded them as the soul, spirit, or quintessence of the plant. Anthroposophists believe they are produced through the action of astral forces in the plant. We understand them as the fragrant principle or the chemical compounds that give a plant its characteristic fragrance. Perhaps it is all four points of view that give scents their magic.

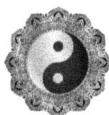

*~ A successful life: to discover your passion
and to be able to creatively express it. ~*

NECTARS, ELIXIRS, AND POTIONS

What is the difference between nectars, elixirs, and potions? By definition they are different, but by design they are very much alike. "Nectar" is derived from the ancient term meaning the "drink of the Gods." A nectar was a sweet nutrient-rich drink, bringing vitality, vigor, and vim to those who drank it.

An elixir is also a sweet-tasting liquid used in compounding medicines. However, it usually contains alcohol. Potions are a little more mystical; usually a beverage made by a magician, sorcerer, dragon, fairy, or witch. It is said to have magical powers. For example, a potion might be made to make a person fall in love with another person. The creation of potions of different kinds was a practice of alchemy and was commonly associated with witchcraft. In the 19th century, it was labeled as "quack medicine," only in later years to be transformed into patented medicines. Today's aspirin is a derivative transformed from an old herbal treatment that included willow bark used to treat headaches.

It is in the mystical world of herbs, aromatherapy, and alchemy that I found the secret and the idea of how to take a nectar, give it a touch of elixir, add a dash of potion, and create, from an ancient idea, a drop of magic that might propel a person to express his or her passion. It takes only a few drops of magic and a little belief to create passionate energy. We all want to feel passion. It is the essential driving force behind all creativity.

Because this book is about sexual health, I'll share with you the story of *Damiana's Nectar*, my sweet nectar that began as a potion, then an elixir, and finally a nectar. But first, I'd like to share with you the process for finding the essence of magic, which is the secret to its power. Here is something from one of my earlier books.

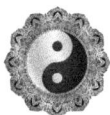

~ A successful life: to watch your children grow up,
get married, and have children. ~

THE QUEST

Our only true desire is to have love and acceptance. Everything else is merely an attempt at obtaining these desires. Men, driven by the desires for love and acceptance, will take their lives to extremes, giving up almost everything for the love of a woman. Throughout the ages, the quest has been to find that one person who would ignite the chemistry of love. We call this the search for our soul mate. It is the purest and most intense essence of love. It is also an aspect of the search for the Philosopher's Stone.

The Philosopher's Stone is not really a stone, but rather a divine and earthly substance from which something relatively worthless is transformed into a precious substance. This substance is the essence of creation. So the story goes, in books from the Bible to the quest for the Holy Grail and written works thereafter, this substance has deep and mysterious secrets. Large volumes of literature throughout history have been written with deeper inner meanings that differ from their outward appearance. One such written work deals with the transmutation of baser metals into gold. This is known as alchemy.

In the days of alchemy (changing form), the alchemists of the Middle Ages sought to transform lead into gold. It was believed that if one could take basic properties and, through a distillation process, remove the impurities, the result would be of divine origin. In the alchemist's view, everything from sand and stones to plants and people had a physical body, a mind, and a soul. The art consisted of distilling the physical body and condensing it into precious substances, the quintessence of life. This is not unlike the laws of karma, where we are directed to cleanse and purify over and over until finally we transcend the birth and death cycles.

Although mystics strove for physical mastery over spiritual wisdom, it was the quest for the divine word of God that predominated alchemy. It was believed that the True Heavenly Stone was in fact the word of God, and that its purpose was to tinge our souls for salvation and eternal life. This divine *word* would lead one to the universal tincture that in fact would turn the ordinary into the extraordinary, but could only be found through the word of God.

The *word*, through its complete understanding of the soul, which it believed should be the only path for those seeking truth, emphasized transmutation of the spirit rather than the physical world. Man was presented as iron in unconverted will and purpose, and it is this, as well as all the thoughts of desire, that must be transmuted into the divine essence.

When reunion between the Creator and creature was accomplished, it was believed the soul would be free of vice, and the heart would be dedicated to virtue and the love of all. The knowledge of God was believed to be the first duty of every reasonable being.

The basic foundation of all things was seen as the spirit of God, and that spirit alone may explain all things. The highest unity was revealed through diversity, and the diversity then must return itself to unity. Ultimately, all is one.

So it is in the quest for love. In the ideal, the souls of a man and woman, through their physical diversity, unify to create the experience of ecstasy and the divine love. Aphrodisiacs of all kinds have been used to bring about this spiritual union. Alchemy of a sort was employed in an attempt to create the pure essence of desire and pleasure. Like the search for the Philosopher's Stone, the alchemist wanted to find a divine and earthly substance from which something relatively worthless is transformed into a precious substance. They did this by simply extracting what is desired to arrive at the essence.

An aphrodisiac is said to arouse sexual desire. The desire for sexual and sensual pleasures is a very powerful urge. Take away the sex drive, and our entire culture would collapse. The drive for power, for money, and the sale of all products and services have a sexual motivation somewhere within the essence. Yes, we would still have the drive of hunger and the need for shelter, but the energy that gives rise to passion and creation would be missing. It is the sexual drive that fuels passion and continues life.

So is it any wonder we have searched endlessly for the essence of desire? After all, it is bliss that keeps the world spinning. Of the seven major emotions that occupy our psyche, the emotions of desire, love, sex, and romance take top billing followed by faith, enthusiasm, and hope.

Within the study of herbs and their historical context, there is a term known as the doctrine of signatures. This refers to the ancient idea that if a plant part in some way resembled a human organ or disease characteristic, that it was useful for that particular organ or ailment.

We need only to look at the pink lady's slipper, asparagus shoots, round- leaved sundew, sweet flag, wood betony, Indian paintbrush, horse nettle, or tulip tree to see the doctrine of signatures. Each of these herbs is purported to be an aphrodisiac.

Herbs and essential oils have been a part of folklore, and thus the substances of love potions throughout history. It should be noted that herbs are plants, and as such, contain vitamins, minerals, and hormones, and it is vitamins, minerals, and hormones that support the sexual drive. This is the magic of herbs. Distill the plants through a process that releases the essence, throw in a little magic, and we get the lifeblood of creation.

Although we think of aphrodisiacs as magical potions, we know that an aphrodisiac is actually a substance that elicits a biochemical response. Sex is really a product of the mind and the brain. It is the petrochemical messages sent by the brain to the rest of the body that cause desire and copulation.

Aphrodisiacs are actually vitamins, minerals, and chemical substances that cause a reaction in the physical, mental, and spiritual self. Herbs and other magic potions are simple organic substances containing the chemicals that ignite the sensual and sexual sensations.

One such herb known to be an aphrodisiac is Damiana. You'll remember from the chapter on herbs that this herb from Mexico and the Southwest has a long and persistent folk history of use as a sexual stimulant. Stress, exhaustion, and excessive living can all lead to a change in mood and low libido. Damiana is nicknamed the "sad mood" herb because it is used to lift a sad mood. Lifting a sad mood has a stimulating effect on the sex brain. Its stimulating properties — starch, sugar, resin, and chlorophyll — are used for nervousness, weakness, and exhaustion and to help clean the blood stream. It is sometimes recommended as an herb that increases sperm count and strengthens ovaries. As a sexual stimulant, it boosts circulation and is a muscle relaxant. All this is conducive to sexual enjoyment. Further, there has been an alkaline that has been identified in Damiana which is said to directly stimulate nerves and sexual organs.

Using the Damiana herb as well as other herbs and ingredients, I developed my mood-enhancing sensuality aphrodisiac, which I named Damiana's Nectar. If you bought the nectar and are now reading this book; or if you're reading the book and contemplating the nectar, here is the true story of its discovery. My discovery of natural aphrodisiacs began with an introduction to an herbal healer. I was searching to find a potion and stumbled upon the recipe for the creation of a nectar that

I named Damiana's Nectar. The following is a true story about adventure, discovery and magic.

It is so true that when the student is ready, the teacher will appear. Several years ago, my world was in a place of adversity and stress. I can now see that this stress was exactly what I needed to begin my journey. Adversity has a way of presenting us with challenge and it is our ability to turn the challenge into creativity that determines the blessings in life. I wanted to find a natural herbal formula to help me cope with the tension, anxiety, and sadness in my life at not being able to find my soul mate. My quest in life was to find my true love. I had been so disappointed by love that I decided to seek out a little help. I had a dream one night that I made a potion and it brought me a great understanding of love. I woke up and began my search by going to the library and reading books on herbs. I found an article in a magazine about a mystical healer who lived about 30 miles north of me. I decided to give her a call.

When I told her about my mission, she spoke with reserve, saying she only saw clients by appointment and was not sure she could help me. With a bit of pleading — and, I believe, a real sincerity on my part — she agreed to meet with me. She gave me specific directions to her home.

I drove the 30 miles, traversing country roads until I came to a row of mailboxes at the end of what appeared to be a driveway. It was marked by an orange sign and an arrow pointing between the bushes. The driveway was a long dirt road that twisted and turned through the middle of an orange grove with the orange trees in full bloom. If you have ever been in California when the orange trees bloom, you know that the air is filled with the sweet smell of citrus. I was swept away by nature's bounty. It was a euphoric drive!

In the center of the grove was a clearing with a small cottage surrounded by gardens of flowers and herbs. On the porch lay two black cats sleeping in the sun. Everything was peaceful.

I opened the door of my car and not a sound could be heard. It was as if I stepped into a fairy tale. The cottage was thatch-roofed with a front porch where two rocking chairs sat completely still in the afternoon sun. Shutters lined the windows and the house was shingled in cedar shakes. It just sat there quietly in the middle of the orange grove. I climbed the steps of the cottage and stood by the door. The inside was shielded only by a wooden screen door. I knocked softly and a woman appeared. She was tall, dressed in black, with long black hair. She was very attractive and smiled warmly as she extended her hand to welcome me into her home.

As I stepped into the little cottage, I noticed the walls were lined with rows of books. The decor was simple, clean, and rustic. She led me through the hallway to her pantry where jars of herbs and potions were neatly organized. From there she led me through a doorway into what appeared to be an office. I sat down, took a deep breath, and it is here in the tranquility of her home that I learned the secret of the nectar of love.

I must admit that in seeking her out, I was not exactly looking for the secret potion of love. What I was really seeking was to find was the part of me that felt empty and alone. As I sat staring at this enchanting woman, I knew at that very moment I was onto something bigger than myself. I knew I was about to embark upon a journey with an unknown destination. I could not turn back. I had to go forward. "What can I help you with?" she asked.

"Well," I cautiously began, "I'm looking for an herbal formula to help me cope with the stress and loneliness in my life. I think everybody struggles with loneliness and I would like to find a magic potion to help. Love has so disappointed me. I am searching for my soul mate. I am searching for love."

She smiled and said, "Perhaps you might want to think about a potion to bring you the essence of love?" She opened a book and read to me, "'There is one basic truth about creation. The world is not inert matter but Gaia, the goddess of living energy. Therefore, the earth and all living things share the same life force and that life force is divine intelligence. All life is an interconnected web. When we honor the earth, the herbs and give praise to the sun and the moon, we align ourselves with the divine intelligence and this unfolds the mysteries of life.'

"Isn't that what you're after?" she asked me. She continued to read, "'Wisdom enriches the soul. It is different from intelligence, information, or knowledge. It reflects an understanding of universal truths. It is based upon an understanding that clarity is not always possible, and that much of life is uncertain. To make a potion you must begin with certain herbs. They must be charged with power before they release their magical essence. You must use your mental energy to act as a catalyst upon the herb's aura. The aura of the herb contains information about the planet that rules its power. Venus, of course, rules love, and so here is where you will find the magical formula for finding true love.'" She took notepaper and wrote down a list of ingredients. "Here," she said, "start with these, and let your intuition be your guide. She then showed me to the door and bid me farewell.

I drove away from the cottage in the middle of the orange grove, down the dusty dirt driveway and back onto the highway. I pulled over to the side of the road and looked at the handwritten formula. It did not have a name, just a list of ingredients and a basic recipe to follow. My heart was pounding, and I was breathless as I realized somewhere within this simple list of ingredients was the secret to the essence of love. I just had to find it.

The basic formula was given to me over 15 years ago. I explored it, I made it, and I improved it. Then I ignored it, improved it, perfected the formula, left it alone, and put it on the shelf. Then one day I took it out, examined it, tasted it, and decided to shares its magic with you. First, let me tell you how the potion became Damiana's Nectar.

The note given to me by my teacher said I should make a simple infusion of herbs. However, before I could make the infusion I needed to read the recipe note again: "learn what you can, take your time, and study the herbs. Potions take time and patience, just like love. The exact formula will not come to you until both you and it are ready. Do not rush these things." Not knowing where to go from here, I went to the library and looked for old books on herbs and folk medicine. After weeks of searching, I came across an old book that had recipes and directions for making infusions, decoctions, tonics, tonic wines, tinctures, elixirs, potions, and nectars. I checked the book out from the library, went home, and devoured it. I made notes and read and reread the book. I renewed it for another two weeks. Then I returned it because I had to give it back for a week before I could take it out again (library rules) in case someone else wanted the book. In two weeks, I returned to take the book out again and I was told that no one could take the book out of the library. It was a book you could use only while in the library. It was a mistake that I was allowed to take the book home. I asked to see the book again and was told that it could not be found. The records showed that I returned the book but after that, it went missing. Luckily for me I had my notes and had written down the steps needed to make a potion.

Armed with the knowledge from the little book and with the recipe from my teacher, I began the process in my kitchen. First, I had to gather the herbs, a linen tea bag, and a Ball canning jar. It takes about a month to distill the formula. The directions I copied from the book read: "Put up on the new moon and draw off on the full moon. Like the tides, the strength of the herb's aura and all of plant life is affected by the gravitational pull of the moon."

So on the first night of the new moon, I charged the herbs by taking the linen tea bag full of the herbal blend into my left hand, closing my eyes and visualizing what I intended the herbs to do. After seeing in my mind's eye the mingling of the aura of the herbs with the aura of my consciousness, I repeated out loud the next step in the recipe, "I ask that this be correct and for the good of all people. So *mote* it be." Meaning — so as I will it, so shall it be done.

I sterilized the jar, filled it with fresh spring water, dropped the herbs in the linen bag inside the jar, sealed the lid of the Ball canning jar, and stashed it away in a dark cool place until the moon was full. Then on the first night of the full moon, I drew off the potion by straining the liquid into a small glass container with a screw-top dropper lid. The potion was sweet with the flavor of the herbs infused into the fresh spring water. The mother potion had been born! Now the problem was that since the potion was in water without some kind of a preservative, it would have a limited shelf life. So I took the mother potion and made it into an elixir, preserving the formula in a base of alcohol. Vodka, to be exact. The taste was strong and bitter. Something was missing. I didn't know what but remembered that the recipe said I should be patient and let the answer come to me. So I bottled it up and put it away on the shelf for about two years. I then began traveling around the country teaching aromatherapy. Through the essence of the oils, I taught others the sensuality of plants or, more notably, the sweet aphrodisiac scents of nature. However, I never gave up my quest for love nor my determination to uncover its secret. So I continued to search for my soul mate and to stay mindful of my herbal potion. As I continued to study the nature of herbal medicine, I found an ancient formula for a "rob," which is a medicinal drink of herbs made into a syrup by adding a sweetener. The sweetener was honey. Honey was used in ancient times for its many medicinal properties and most notably to help the "medicine go down." Eureka! It suddenly came to me. The answer! Add honey, and my elixir became a nectar, the sweet drink of the gods, namely Venus. Now add a little natural flavoring such as chocolate (an aphrodisiac) and Damiana's Nectar was born!

But now, the problem was how to make it, bottle it, and label it. At the time, I was consulting with a small supplement company and mentioned my dilemma to one of my associates. She introduced me to the man who was manufacturing their products, suggesting he might know someone to help me. He, in turn, introduced me to a manufacturer who knew exactly what I wanted and how to produce the formula from my mother potion. At the same time I met a young woman who came to my yoga class and wanted to have private yoga lessons but could not afford my fee, so she offered to design a label for me in exchange. It all suddenly came together, but I did not have the money to produce and market the formula. I had to shelve it again for another few years.

Then I met my now husband. After twenty-five years of searching, I met my soul mate but not without employing a little magic. And now, here I sit sharing this all with you, producing the formula and releasing Damiana's Nectar; the nectar of love.

I was given the formula for the nectar of love. It was meant to be shared. It has been charged with the power of the moon and blessed by the planet Venus. The secret is not really a secret, but like all things within its context is a deeper hidden meaning that will only reveal itself to you when you are ready to receive. If you follow closely you will uncover the hidden meaning. But use caution, because you should use the magic you discover only for the happiness and good of all. When it comes to matters of the heart, kindness, respect, appreciation, and understanding will always bring you love. However, adding a little magic never hurts!

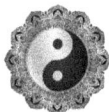

*~ A successful life: to appreciate beauty
and find the best in others. ~*

LIGHT, COLOR, AND MUSIC –
VIBRATION HEALTH

S ince the beginning of time, light has been an integral
part of creation and evolution. Sunlight, our source
of warmth and energy, sustains all life on Earth. It
sustains the earth itself. It provides plants with the energy
for photosynthesis, providing food, water, and oxygen for
plants, insects, animals, and humans. It is through light
that we are able to see. The sun sends electromagnetic
waves of energy to the earth with only a small amount
reaching the earth. The eye is believed to perceive only
about 1% of these electromagnetic waves. The
percentage it perceives contains the colors of the rainbow
from violet (the shortest wavelength) to red (the longest
wavelength). Seeing is a very important aspect of human
evolution and functioning. Our health, our well-being,
and our lives are dependent upon the light of the sun.
Think about the transition of colors from dawn to dusk.
What are the various physiological and psychological

moods you transition through as the light and colors around you change? Ever noticed what happens when you go out in the country and surround yourself with the light of the sun and the colors of nature? Tranquility often transpires — the blood pressure lowers, stress is relieved, the heart rate and pulse slow, and our moods improve.

Exposure to sunlight influences humans in a variety of ways. Two of the best known are fertility and mood. In northern-hemisphere countries, studies have shown that a disorder called seasonal affective disorder (SAD) affects a good percentage of the population and that, in the cold winter months where there is a lower exposure to sunlight, a higher degree of irritability, fatigue, illness, insomnia, depression, alcoholism, and suicide have been present.

The therapeutic use of light and color has been documented for thousands of years. Albert Szent-Györgyi, Nobel Prize winner and the discoverer of vitamin C, concluded that all the energy we take into our bodies is derived from the sun. Human beings are nourished directly by sunlight and indirectly by eating foods, drinking liquids, and breathing air that has been vitalized by the sun's energy. Since light has a profound effect on everything and our eyes are the mechanism for processing light and color and bringing it directly to the brain, it would appear that the eyes are more than just something for "seeing."

This book is about natural sexual health. Light, color, and music are elements in the dance of sexual love. We need to go back to biochemistry in order to truly understand how light and color affects our sexual selves. Sunlight enters the eyes and activates the pineal gland — which is believed to be responsible for regulating the body's biological clock or its rhythms, when to wake up, and when to sleep. The pineal accomplishes this rhythmic feat by messages it receives from the hypothalamus, which tells the pineal when to release melatonin, a compound that circulates through living organisms.

Melatonin is released in response to darkness with a peak release about 2:00 AM – 3:00 AM. Melatonin is secreted directly into the blood and can be found everywhere in the body. Now it is widely accepted that animals living in the natural environment breed on a seasonal basis, and the amount of light they see determines the reproductive status. Each species requires a certain amount of light in order to remain sexually competent and melatonin helps us to regulate our physical activity based upon light and darkness. Melatonin affects our moods and energy levels by regulating our circadian rhythms. Rest, mood, and energy positively affect our sexual desires and performances.

In a study conducted at Boston State Hospital, Dr. Abraham Myerson found that ultraviolet light increased male sex hormones by 120%, and increased the female sex hormone, estrogen, as well. What we can conclude from this is that light has a profound effect on animal mating and reproduction.

Light energy interacts with all of life. If light energy should come to a halt, it would have devastating consequences. However, these consequences go deeper than the destruction of the physical world. Beneath the visible world is what physicists call the subatomic world. Physicists tell us that all of life is composed of energy and radiation. This reinforces what many believe: that physical things radiate energy. This energy is called the aura. It is a vibration of energy fields that emits from everything. Science further explains energy to be light that is beyond the naked human eye. The aura is a vibration of energy that is integral to human beings and all of life.

Think about a time when you were in nature and felt the soothing calmness that radiated from the plant life and the bodies of water. When we travel to tranquil places our energy field gets harmonized first and then our bodies begin to relax and harmonize with the environment.

Once you feel the energy and begin to relax, the body and the mind soon follow.

What this all means is we all have an aura, and part of the flowing energy of that aura is sensual and sexual. This is the part of the aura we are the most interested in enhancing. What we need to remember is that the light of the aura fractures into the colors red, orange, yellow, green, blue, indigo, and violet. It is much like a prism where light leaving the prism disperses and refracts the white light into its component color rays. These colors all have energy levels that can be measured in wavelengths and vibrations. So, not only does light have a profound effect upon us, but the various colors that make up the white light also affect us. The best example of this would be to take us back out in nature where we are mostly surrounded with the color green. On the color spectrum, green is the middle color or the balancing center. If we are in touch with our energy when in a green natural environment, we'll feel a sense of balance and calmness. Green is strong and centering and yet soothing in an energetic way.

Now remember that light energy stimulates the pineal gland, and light energy is made up of a band of colors all vibrating at different frequencies. These different frequencies have different vibrations that affect us in different ways. What we really want to know is how to take our sensual and sexual selves to an enhanced vibration level. Let us look at a brief description of the effects of the seven colors of the rainbow. If you wish to know more about color and light energy, go to colourenergy.com ask for Maria. Tell her Doctor Lynn sent you.

Light is made up of colors, and these colors have an effect upon the natural world. Let us take a brief look at color and color therapy.

Red stimulates, excites, and warms the body. It increases heart rate, brain wave activity, and respiration. Red is the color associated with the first chakra or energy center connected with our aura or vibrating energy. Red and its energy represent instinct, survival, habits, and ordinary day-to-day life.

Orange, the second color center, is associated with stimulating the nerves of the sex organs. When this energy is balanced, a person has flair and is expressive. It is essential that this color center be balanced to enhance sexual health. Orange also stimulates appetite and reduces fatigue. Think about orange if you want to cook a sexy meal and rev up your lover. Think pumpkin pie with a sprinkle of cinnamon...

Yellow is for memory. It is also the color of sunshine so it is energizing and lifts depression. Yellow represents power and the ability to focus. If this color is not in balance, a person has a tendency to become overly emotional, intense, and passionate. In balance, a person finds strength and will power.

Green, remember, is the color that gives us balance and is the center of our being. It connects to the heart and, when in balance, is said to fill us with love and expansion. You begin to realize through the green color center what it means to sacrifice for the sacrifice and to love without conditions. If green is weak, there is a tendency to overextend, feel overwhelmed, and lack compassion. Green is the most prominent color on earth. Green is an excellent color when dieting; bring green into your diet, exercise, and spiritual life and watch what happens!

Blue is cooling, especially in a hot and humid environment. Blue has a cooling and calming effect on the body-mind. It lowers respiration and heart rate. It is the color of creativity and communication. Our love and our passion can freely be expressed when this center is in balance. If stuck, we experience blocked creativity and have difficulty being direct.

Indigo is said to "pierce the veil of illusion," and open the body-mind to awareness and focus. When this color energy center is in balance, our intuitive sense is strengthened. You know when you feel that unspoken sense of attraction. It is the blue/indigo energy doing its stuff! Indigo also affects the emotional self by making one calmer and more inward-thinking.

Violet is said to belong to the soul or the higher consciousness. Violet is uplifting in a spiritual sense. It vibrates at 731 trillion times per second, making it invisible to the naked eye at this vibration level. It is believed to be the color that takes us beyond the ordinary and into ecstasy.

All of these colors then blend back into white light, which is the purest of all. The theory of color therapy is based upon the physical, mental, and spiritual effects of light and color. Remember, light is transferred to the hypothalamus where it is interpreted by the pituitary and pineal glands and then communicated to the body-mind. There are numerous health-related uses for light and color. This book is about enhancing your sex life, so all the wonders of color and light cannot be covered. Again, try www.colourenergy.com and ask for Maria for more information on light and color therapy.

For now, just remember the colors of the spectrum, and that light and color have a profound effect on our health and, thus, our sexual health. In addition, one more thing:

as well as light and color have vibration energy that affects us, sounds also can affect our energy. Think about a love song and how it makes you feel. What happens to your body and your emotions as you switch from one type of music to another? Put on a march like *March Militaire* by Schubert or *Mars* from the Gustav Holst's *The Planets Suite*. Observe your body-mind and how the vibration of the music affects you.

It has been theorized that the sound of the mother's heartbeat, being the first sound a human hears, is the doorway to consciousness. Sound is the first sense to awaken. The rhythmic beat of drums has been used to induce transcendental states. Ticking alarm clocks are sometimes used to sooth puppies that have been removed from their mother. Sound, of course, brings us music, and music, it seems, is more than simply a distraction. Studies show that music can actually give you a better aerobic workout and a better strength-training workout. Those working out to music pumped more iron and burned more calories than a study group that exercised without music.

Music puts us in the mood. Sounds make their way through the ear canal into the limbic system where the vibration causes a variety of basic instincts and emotional cues to happen. You know what it is like when you feel the beat and just have to get up and dance!

Hospitals, prisons, schools, malls, and workplaces are all using light, color, and sound to enhance the environment for healing, calming, working, and relaxing. Awareness of the world around you — especially sight, sound, smell, touch, taste, and intuition — is the key to living a sexy life.

\

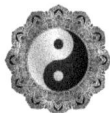

~ A successful life: to feel a kiss, a hug,
and smell the scent of and taste someone you love. ~

SENSUALITY OF SEX – TASTE, SMELL, TOUCH, SOUND, SIGHT, AND INTUITION

Webster's Dictionary defines sensuality as being of the body and the senses, as distinguished from the intellect. It further describes it as being connected or preoccupied with sexual pleasures. Since *sensuality* means "of the senses," it would seem that if one were a sensual being, then the sensations received through all the senses are humanity's gifts to enjoy.

Sensuality sells! It is the mystique and the allure of the pleasures of the senses that is behind a majority of the products and services provided. Everyone wants to be sexy, alluring, exciting, wanted, and pursued. This is the promise of most of the products we see advertised. If only it was as easy as buying a car, a perfume, a dress or taking a vacation.

To ignite the fires of passion, it takes a buffet of elements, including hormones, the senses, intimacy, love, passion, attraction, mood, and affection. However, the senses bring the experience of human ecstasy into existence. Without the senses, it is impossible to have the human experience (as we know it) of lovemaking and of life.

Our sexual, biological self is a physiological response as opposed to the response of the senses. The senses excite us, sending messages to the brain to ignite the hormonal response. Sensuality is of the senses and sexuality is biochemical. The two together create pleasure and delight.

So, if it is the sensual experience that brings pleasure to humans, then it would seem that we should be able to enhance the senses through various methods found in nature. Without the sensory experience of sight, sound, touch, smell, taste, and intuition, how could we experience the gift of life?

Sensuality means the senses are engaged! There is no denying that the senses must be heightened for the process of sexuality to take place. For animals, it is the sense of smell that determines the mating process, but for us humans it is a bit more complex.

Scientists believe that as the brain evolved, higher primates such as human beings, began to rely more on the sense of sight to determine attraction. It is true that we live in a visual world, and it is also true that men are more visual than women. Although sight is what first attracts us, the sound of one's voice either keeps us interested or quickly extinguishes the desire. Everyone has had the experience of seeing an attractive person and the minute they open their mouth, the tone of the voice, the pitch, and the quality of the message will either make or break the initial attraction.

If we get past the sight and sound, the smell, touch, and taste cement the deal! With all the senses in full swing we are hooked, addicted, and full tilt into the sensual experience. But how do the senses work, and what can we do to enhance the experience of sensuality?

You'll recall from a few paragraphs back, scientists believe that, as humans evolved, the sense of sight became the determining factor of attraction over the sense of smell, the primary factor of attraction in lower primate animals. Remember, that as the human brain evolved, the sexual response engaged higher levels of the human brain known as the limbic system and the cerebral cortex.

For you to be aware of or to sense your external and internal environments there must be some kind of stimulus. Sensory receptors are the body's communication channels, receiving stimuli from both the outside and the inside world. The body has a mosaic of neural receptors, which direct stimuli such as pain, temperature, and touch. The body also has special receptors, which detect smell, light, sound, and taste.

Impulses (energy) conducted to specific sensory areas of the cerebral cortex produce conscious sensations. Only the cerebral cortex can see a sexy person, hear a sexy voice, and feel a sexy body. In other words, the true sensation takes place in our heads!

Deep within the body in the walls of the blood vessels and organs are the internal sense receptors. They tell us when we are hungry, thirsty, horny, sick, or tired. The receptors sensitive to outside stimuli are located near the body's surface. They allow us to see, hear, feel, taste, and smell. It is the outside sensations that send sensual messages to the brain.

The receptors near the body's surface that sense changes in the external environment and affect our sense of touch, pain, pressure, and vibration are called the general senses. The special senses of seeing, smelling, tasting, and hearing are much more specialized and complex. Hearing receptors sense sound waves, whereas taste and smell receptors sense chemicals.

As we grow and change, so do our senses and sensory perceptions. Our sense of self and our sense of the world are constantly in a state of flux. Memory plays a key role in retaining sensory experience, as well as the physical and mental process of organizing the information into recognizable patterns.

As far as we know, we come into this world with five senses, and each of those plays an intricate role in our sensuality and sexuality. Let us take a look at each of the senses of pleasure!

Through the intimate embrace of lovemaking, we literally engage all the senses. We see, smell, taste, touch, and hear our lover. Without the total engagement of the senses, we would not be able to experience the depth of passion. You might say, "Well, what about a person who can't see or hear their lover?" It is well known that when one of the senses is missing, the other senses intensify. One can "see" through the sense of touch, smell, or taste; and one can "hear" through the sense of sight or touch by watching or feeling body language.

We live in a visual world. Within five seconds of meeting someone, we are either attracted or not. Sight is probably the first indicator of sexual attraction. It is the stimulus that causes us to approach a person. For men the visual cues are the first indicator of attraction and arousal.

Women are a bit more complicated. However, sight alone is not enough to keep us interested and to bind us sexually to another person.

Once we approach another person, the sound of their voice is often the next cue to our attraction level. We use the sense of hearing to draw conclusions about a person. The tone of the voice and the manner of speaking either draw us deeper into the attraction mode or quickly make the attraction fade. Sound waves and the vibration tone have a profound effect upon our sexual attraction. Think about a time you either fell in love with a voice or found the sound so discordant you recoiled. That is the power of sound.

If we get past sight and sound, touch is the next sense to take control. The touch of a person can be a very powerful binding agent. We know that oxytocin, a powerful peptide, can bind two people together. A touch, a hug, and a kiss — if enjoyed — can lead to sex.

The kiss brings with it the sense of taste, and the hug brings a sense of smell. Although these senses are not the most prominent, science knows that through pheromones and body chemistry that taste and smell also create a strong reaction.

The five senses work together to create the chemistry of attraction, lust, and love. Without attraction through the senses, typical sexual encounters would never happen. Of course, sexual encounters can happen without any level of attraction. However, even at an animalistic level of sexuality there must be some kind of sensual stimulation.

Sensuality is the essence of sexuality. When tuned into sex, we become excited through the sensual self. We see, hear, touch, smell, and taste our lover. As I am writing this chapter, I just finished speaking with someone who is having virtual sex over the Internet with someone she has never met in real life. He is a cartoon character with a perfect body, features, and looks. She has fallen for and been intimate with someone she has never seen, touched, heard, smelled, or tasted. Her sensory world has been excited by the keystrokes of the computer and an imaginary fantasy world where everyone is perfect.

Does this mean we can now have sexual relationships without any physical contact? If being turned on to sex means being excited and stimulated through the sexual self, how can we become so involved with computer games and pornography sites? We see what we want to see, and we hear what we want to hear, and imagination and our fantasy world create stimuli for the senses. After all, in real life or in fantasy, the excitement of sex is oftentimes the imagined and not the real. It's that elusive side of fantasy that resides in our heads.

Even with computer technology and cyber sex, the senses are still stimulated because it is the power of attraction and imagination inside the brain that keeps us ignited and involved. Infatuation and imagination are powerful tools. They make the reality of everyday life a fantasy. However, the senses get dull and the return to reality leaves a void in the deep sensual experience of making love. Remember Pygmalion and the statue? Perfection does not always mean love and sensual joy. For me, I'll take the reality of the sensual experience over voyeurism and fantasy, where all my senses are engaged and love has a chance to flourish.

The most basic element of human sexual response is for procreation. It is through sex that we perpetuate the species. Nature has endowed the universe with sensual aids to ensure the procreation of nature.

However, the human element is far more complex. We have feelings, expectations, and desires, and of all the pleasures of life, our sensual expression is the most profound.

Beyond the physical pleasure, human sexuality serves as an important reinforcement of pair bonding between two individuals. This is what separates humans from the rest of the animal kingdom.

We know that deterioration of health plays a part in our ability to continue to enjoy sex. However, if we are physically active, healthy, strong, and alert, we can enjoy sex well past midlife. The key is to be healthy. Drugs and surgery will not make us healthy; neither will artificial stimulants like Viagra. However, proper nutrition, exercise, rest, play, and the right attitude are what have the power to make us healthy, happy, and vibrant.

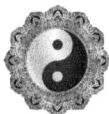

~ A successful life: to leave the world a better place. ~

XERCISE FOR A SEXY BODY & MIND

According to the *Journal of the American Medical Association* (JAMA), from a study released in 1999, about 43% of women and about 31% of men suffer sexual inadequacy for one reason or another. While the study did not look at specific causes of dysfunction, it did conclude that many of the dysfunctions were treatable. One such treatment is exercise. Researchers found that exercise increases blood flow and circulation to all parts of the body, including the genital organs. The researchers found that those who exercise regularly have higher levels of desire, greater sexual confidence and frequency, and an enhanced ability to be aroused and achieve orgasm — no matter what their age! Aerobics, strength training, and yoga all release endorphins in the brain, the biochemical that makes us feel good.

A good workout makes for a better body image and the simple act of exercising, regardless of your weight or fitness level, can make you feel positive about how you look and how you perform. Whether it be sexual, athletic, or everyday energy output, performance is important. Having strength, endurance, stamina, and quick recovery time as well as a positive state of mind are all conducive to winning in the game of love.

A University of Washington study found that 20 minutes of cycling enhanced sexual arousal by 169% in women. There are many exercises including yoga, swimming, and dancing that can enhance our sex lives by elevating energy, stamina, passion, and pleasure.

But did you know that 20 minutes of good sex can burn up to 160 calories and one long, passionate kiss can burn 12 calories? Regular sex is good for the body, mind, and soul. Scientific research has shown that regular sex improves circulation, heart rate, flexibility, breathing, weight control, and attitude. Touching, hugging, kissing, and loving all produce those "feel good" hormones flooding the body-mind with a sense of calm and pleasure. Some of the benefits of regular sex are better sleep, reduced stress, increased self-esteem, and pain relief. And it makes us smile! We are happier, healthier, and sharper!

Some major blocks to experiencing good sex (given we are healthy and able) are stress and lack of physical strength, endurance, and flexibility. Exercise removes these blocks. Therefore, *SEX-ercising* should be part of a program to enhance sexual health. That's why I developed Doctor Lynn's Xercise for a Sexy Body-Mind. You can do the entire program live over the Internet with me each week. There will be great music to get you up and moving. Go to my website for details. Also a short video of my Xercise program can be downloaded to your computer from my website. Here, I will give you the first part of the three-part class in written form. Please note that some of the exercises are yoga exercises, stretching exercises and exercises specifically to open and strengthen the pelvic region in both men and women. Parts two and three are taught live in my studio and over the Internet.

Doctor Lynn's Xercise for a Sexy Body-Mind strengthens, opens, flexes and relaxes the sexual muscles of the body and the mind. For now, simply follow this simple set of exercises to enhance your body and mind. The secret to great sex is not found in positions but in a healthy self that is balanced, flexible, strong, and happy. Breathing is essential to exercise and to good sex, so pay attention to the breathing techniques. Follow the breath as it moves about your body.

Find a quiet, warm place. Place your mat, blanket, or towel on the floor. Lie down on your back with your knees bent. Place your right hand on your heart and your left hand on your sacral or pelvic area between your hipbones. Inhale deeply through your nose, into your heart, and exhale out through your nose and your abdomen. Just experience the rise of the breath in your chest and the fall of the breath in your belly. When the heart center is out of balance, we are closed off from love. We lack compassion and understanding. We find it difficult to say no and can become overwhelmed with emotion. We can become hardhearted. When the sacral center is out of balance, we become overly obsessed with sex or totally cut off from our sexual energy. Now, take in five deep breaths, breathing into the heart and out through the sacral.

Stand up for posture strength. Think about sex appeal. Nothing says sex appeal like good posture and a sexy walk. Standing Mountain pose makes us aware of our posture. It stretches and elongates the spine, opens the chest, and improves breathing. It is a centering pose that helps us to achieve balance. Standing Mountain reminds us that to stand tall as the mountain is to stand with confidence and strength. Ever heard that self-confidence is sexually alluring? Stand up straight. Feel your feet pressed into the mat; balls and heels of feet pushing evenly. Pull in your abdominal muscles, lift up through your chest, pull your shoulders back, and take in a deep breath. Take in four more breaths

Squats. Standing, place your hands on your hips and straighten your legs. Now bend your knees and squat.

Then pull back up, straightening the knees and squeeze the pelvic area and the buttocks. Bend again and repeat eight times. On the eighth one, pull up, hold the pose, tighten the buttocks muscle, place your hands on your buttocks and squeeze as tightly as you can, holding for a count of four. Release and relax with a deep inhale and exhale. This will strengthen your legs, hips, and buttocks, which is good for sex!

Pelvic/abdominal squeeze. Stand with your feet about 12 inches apart. Slightly bend your knees and place your hands on your thighs. Center your pelvic area. As you inhale, tighten the pelvic muscles between your legs and draw the breath up and under the rib cage. Now exhale back out down through the abdomen and out through the pelvic area. Do this five times. This exercise will strengthen the PC muscles, which are essential to good sex. It will also strengthen the diaphragm to improve breathing, another essential ingredient to having good sex.

Kegels. Kegels exercises are necessary to support sexual endurance and enjoyment. The reason for kegels exercises is to strengthen the pubococcygeus (PC) also known as the "love muscle" which helps both men and women have strong and lasting orgasms. Age, pregnancy, and lack of sexual activity can weaken these muscles, causing urinary incontinence, premature ejaculation, lack of a firm erection, lack of lubrication, and inability to orgasm. Therefore, strong PC muscles enhance erections and orgasms in both men and women. The easiest way to find the PC muscles is to stop the flow of urine in midstream. When you squeeze you are working the PC muscles. However, once you locate them, you should do this as an exercise and not while urinating. Squeeze as if you are urinating and the phone rings and you need to hold it to answer the phone. The PC muscles, like any other muscle in the body, must be "worked out." If they become weak, sex suffers. I would recommend doing these daily. My *Doctor Lynn's Anti-Aging* DVD also has a section devoted to strengthening the PC. You can find it on my website.

Pelvic lift. Lie on your back with your knees bent. Lift your buttocks/hips up toward the ceiling. Lift as high as you can and then squeeze your buttocks and abdominal muscles. Release by bringing your buttocks back down to the floor. Do this 10 times. Always pull your pelvic area up as far as possible, squeeze tightly, and then release back down to the mat. The pelvic tilt strengthens your hips, thighs, and buttocks. It gives you strength to lift and push, which happens to be a good thing when it comes to sex!

Kegel crunches. Move down on your back with knees bent. Cup your hands together behind your head. Lift your buttocks off the mat, squeeze the PC muscles and then lift your head and hold for a count of four. Release back to the mat. Repeat eight times.

Butterfly. Rest on your back. Bend your knees and bring the soles of your feet together. Let your knees drop open (keeping the soles of the feet together) and hold for about 10 seconds. Bring the knees back up and together and squeeze the PC. Repeat this eight times. Then drop the knees open and hold for 10 seconds. This exercise will open the pelvic area and is beneficial for urinary problems, which can get in the way of good sex. Stopping halfway through sex to go to the bathroom sure breaks the mood!

Rope climb. Straighten your legs and lie flat on the mat. Stretch your arms straight up towards the ceiling over your chest area. Lift your head and shoulders off the mat and move your arms as if you are climbing up a rope. Do this for a count of 10. Rest and repeat three more times. This will strengthen your core and abdominal muscles, as well as arms and shoulders. It will also help you reach and hold your lover with strength and passion.

Cobra pose. Roll over on your stomach with your arms at your sides and your chin resting on the mat. Bring your arms up onto your back and clasp the hands together. Pull the shoulders up and back and, at the same time, lift your head and look straight ahead. Inhale as you lift and exhale as you release back down to the mat. Repeat three more times. Cobra strengthens and adds flexibility to the upper back while strengthening the belly. Cobra also focuses on strengthening the sacrum or pelvic area, which in yoga, is the seat of sexuality. Keep your back strong because you never know when you'll find yourself on your back!

Stick pose. Sit straight with your legs extended out. Place your hands at your hips and pull yourself up so you feel your sit bones pushing into the mat. Straighten your spine and sit tall. Flex your feet back as far as you can. You will feel a stretch in your legs that extends up to your hips. Stick pose works the sexual nerves from the tip of the toes all the way up the spine. Hold and breathe for five long breaths. This pose will strengthen your hips and is said to help with sexual dysfunction. Strong legs and hips help us to wrap around our lover in provocative ways.

Leg lifts. Sit up and bring the soles of your feet together. Place your hands on your feet, lower your head and shoulders and take in three deep breaths. Now sit up and stretch your legs straight out in front of you. Place your arms behind you to support your weight. Lift your feet and legs a few inches off the mat and swing them open. Pull them back while bending the knees and pulling the knees in toward the chest. Extend the legs back out and repeat 10 times. Inhale and exhale on each movement. This exercise works the sex nerves by rhythmically opening and closing the hip and pelvic area. And we know what happens when we rhythmically move those hips!

Arm extensions. Sit up and cross your legs. Stretch arms out at shoulder height. Make a fist by pulling your fingers into the mound of your hand with your thumbs pointing straight up. As you inhale, roll your thumbs back, then exhale, and roll your thumbs straight up. Inhale and roll your thumbs forward and then exhale and roll your thumbs straight up. Repeat 4 times. Then bend your elbows and roll the thumbs in towards your shoulders and then back out. Repeat 4 times. This exercise strengthens the arms and shoulders as well as stimulates the pituitary gland, which releases feel-good neurochemicals that enhance the sexual part of our brain. Balancing the hemispheres of the brain is said to balance emotions. Emotional balance allows you to let go and concentrate on the task at hand.

Open plexus. Roll over onto your back. Sit up and bend your knees and lean back resting onto your elbows supporting your lower back with your hands. Take a deep breath and drop your head and shoulders back with a slight arch to the back, opening the plexus/sexual center. Breathe three long, deep breaths and relax. Here you are opening up the lower nerve plexus, releasing any sexual blocks and connecting with your sexual essence.

The plexus center is a network of intersecting nerves. They combine and connect with spinal nerves, creating a network. There are several networks in the body, including the sacral plexus, which stimulates the pelvis, buttocks, genitals, thighs, calves, and feet.

Relax. Drop your body to the mat with your legs stretched out. Place your right hand over your heart and your left hand over your sacral. Close your eyes and breathe into your heart and out through your sacral. When the heart center is balanced, we experience love, expansion and a lifted spirit. We love without condition. When the sacral is balanced we are open, expressive. We give and we receive. Take in five deep breathes; breathing in through the heart and out through the sacral. Then relax and take a few moments to release your sexual energy.

Come up to a sitting position, cross your legs, and place your hands on your knees. Close your eyes and take in a deep breath and release. Just sit quietly and experience your sexual essence.

Your sexuality and your well-being are the foundation of your life. So carry this energy with you and live well.

Vibration energy in the heart and sacral centers has an effect on our sexual energy. Exercise helps us to strengthen and open these important energy centers. Exercise combined with music and color as well as diet, herbs, nectars, and scents will enhance our sexual energy.

After you have done the above Doctor Lynn's Xercise routine, it is time to participate in an aerobic activity. Aerobic exercise gets the blood flowing and activates those brain chemicals called endorphins. Study after study has shown that exercise enhances health, and more specifically, sexual health. Feeling good in both body and mind is a great aphrodisiac. I would suggest joining me for parts two and three of Doctor Lynn's Xercise for a Sexy Body- Mind. For more information go to my website www.doctorlynn.com. If you cannot get to a class, join me online in the virtual gym where we'll dance and have fun! If you prefer walking, download from my website a playlist of fun songs guaranteed to get you moving. Here is a playlist of 12 songs I just love. Visit my website each month and you will find a new playlist compiled by my students and me.

Download these tunes from iTunes or any other music site onto your iPod or computer:

- *Take Me to the Clouds Above/Radio Edit*
- *Ohh La La/Goldfrappe*

- *Cosmic Love/Florence and the Machine 4. Control/Dataworx*
- *Bad Moon on the Rise/Credence Clearwater 120*
- *I Can't Go for That/The Bird and the Bee*
- *Vanishing Point/Apollo 440*
- *Whataya Want from Me/Adam Lambert*
- *My Girl/Temptations*
- *Seventeen/Lady Tron*
- *Let It Be /Benny Benassie*
- *We Like to Party/Vengaboys*

Sound and movement are among the fundamental ritualistic practices of modern humans. What other living thing listens to music and reflects, escapes, dreams, dances, and is moved to ecstasy by sound, rhythm, the vibration, and the beat as it penetrates the body-mind. Dance is as old as civilization. Humans dance to life, at weddings, births, parties, and the sowing and reaping of our bounties. Dance is something all romantic lovers do. Sexual excitement can be found in movement and the flirtatious dance of attraction. So get up and dance!

The Doctor Lynn's Xercise for a Sexy Body-Mind video with accompanying music will allow you to simultaneously get in touch with the movement of your body and the stillness of your mind. Practice it at least three times a week. The days in between, listen to your own playlist, take a walk, join a class, dance, and have fun.

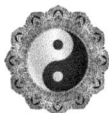

~ A successful life: to give something of you
that helps another person grow. ~

THE MIND IS A SEXY THING

It has been said that the mind is the greatest aphrodisiac of all. Sexual attraction begins in the mind. It happens deep within our thoughts long before we actually make the physical move. Ever felt that angst of sexual tension with someone you do not even know? How about someone at the gym that you see every day but have never spoken with...however, you feel the sexual attraction. It is all in the mind's eye!

There is one sure thing that will kill sexual attraction and that is negativity. Probably the number one killer is depression, followed by anger. Depression is responsible for a good portion of our sexual dysfunction. It dulls sensuality and can leave us feeling lethargic, empty, and lonely.

Everyone experiences bouts of sadness and depression. Usually they are mild and self-limiting. However, specific biochemical changes in the brain can be observed during sadness and depression. Stress, low self-esteem, anxiety, aging, and loss of sexual functioning can all be causes of sadness and depression. However, more than just the mood inside our body's chemistry is at work. Our moods, just like our energy and our health, are affected by the biochemistry of our entire being.

When you hear of depression, you usually think of someone crying and apathetic. But in truth, many people who are depressed don't show outward signs. Usually they are feeling sad, agitated, or anxious. When they bring these symptoms to their doctors, they are prescribed antidepressants, which may have an adverse affect on their sexuality. Regarding our sexual health, this can create a vicious cycle. Depression happens. Libido drops, sex stops, and we miss the touching, loving, and pleasure of orgasm. Then depression deepens. Now, this does not mean that if a person is severely depressed that they should not seek out medical help. It simply means that we should also look to our diet and lifestyle habits when it comes to limiting depression. Biochemistry plays an important role in our sexual and overall health.

It is interesting to note that the same vitamins and minerals that uplift our moods also enhance our sexual energy. For example, the B vitamins are known to be helpful with lifting depression. These same B vitamins support sexual health. Because the diet influences the brain's behavior, it's important to eat healthy whole foods and avoid empty-calorie fast foods and snack foods. The neurotransmitters dopamine, serotonin, and norepinephrine regulate our behavior through the foods we eat. When serotonin is produced, we tend to be more relaxed and tension is eased. Dopamine and norepinephrine cause us to act more quickly and to be more alert and uplifted. The substance that produces serotonin is the amino acid tryptophan. Complex carbohydrates such as fruits, vegetables, and whole grains raise the level of tryptophan in the brain, causing a calming effect. Protein promotes dopamine and norepinephrine production, which promotes alertness. So, consume more carbohydrates than protein if you are nervous and wish to relax and more protein if you are tired and want to become more alert. Therefore, to put your sexual self in the right frame of mind, start with a healthy diet.

Another important vitamin to keep the brain healthy and happy is vitamin "T," or the touch vitamin. We crave touch. Touch makes us feel good. It soothes anxiety and depression because it releases oxytocin, the feel-good peptide. When we are caressed, oxytocin gives us that warm and sensual feeling. Oxytocin increases dopamine, making us feel giddy, and serotonin, making us feel relaxed. Estrogen, touch, and sexual intercourse increase oxytocin. The body softens with touch, the brain releases feel-good neurochemicals and the mind gets playful and aroused.

Vitamin "V," or vasopressin, is also a peptide that helps the mind feel good and sexy. Oxytocin makes us feel giddy and forgetful while vasopressin provides a nice balance by making us focus. It enhances our attention and alertness in the here and now. Vasopressin is also active in the orgasmic (septal) part of our brain, setting both the emotional and physical thermostat. Vasopressin is a brain hormone involved with memory, learning, and recall. It causes us to want to be monogamous and discourages emotional extremes. Vasopressin also plays an important part in our sleep patterns, which affect our mental attitudes. Sleep deprivation plays havoc on our sex lives. We need adequate amounts of REM sleep — the dream stage — to maintain emotional stability. When we have excessively emotional dreams, the brain cuts off REM sleep to prevent the body from overheating. Vasopressin is the neurotransmitter that causes this to happen. It balances out our emotional states. A balanced emotional state is a lot sexier than a tired, wildly emotional, irritable, depressed lover. Vasopressin also influences our brain waves, and brain waves influence our sexual health.

The brain is powered by electricity and produces brain waves. There are four brain waves: beta, alpha, theta, and delta. Beta activity is associated with alertness, arousal, and concentration; alpha with relaxation; theta with creativity, memory, integrative experiences, and healing; and delta with sleep, profound rest, and release of the growth hormone. Theta is known as the twilight state or the dreamlike state we experience just before we fall asleep. During both orgasm and REM sleep, the brain generates theta brain waves. Vasopressin is produced in both REM sleep and theta activity. Remember, vasopressin balances out our emotions, allowing us to maintain a deeper REM sleep where sexual cues are stored. During REM sleep, men get nocturnal erections and women lubricate. Dopamine increases the flow of vasopressin; so by boosting the flow of our body's natural euphoria, dopamine, we can increase the flow of vasopressin, generate theta activity, be more relaxed and emotionally balanced, and produce both erections and lubrication. I would say that is a good thing! How do we accomplish this? Touch, hug, relax, get a good night's sleep, and stay focused on the here and now.

The ideal would be to take two people and blend this cocktail of monogamy and excitability. Two people in synch have the ability to get onto the "same wavelength." If you have ever been totally in harmony with another person, you know what I mean. It is a pleasurable ride where communication flows and the mind is uplifted and focused. When we are together on the same wavelength, communication is open and expressive, inhibitions are dropped, and the sexual messages are deep and flowing. When you are in the same brain-mind state as your lover, the experience is enhanced. If you have experienced deep lovemaking, you have experienced this state of sexual communication. The brain produces the bits of information, and the mind organizes it into thoughts and emotions. The mind acts upon these messages, the body engages, and love is made.

For now, it is enough to understand that when we are in the same mind state, our shared experience is amplified. The mind decides what is pleasurable and what is not. The mind also receives messages from the senses, which receive messages from the natural and unnatural world. How these messages are interpreted is up to the individual. Beauty, after all, is in the mind of the beholder. On the other hand, think of it this way: it is the mind that "sees" the sunset. The eyes let in the light, color, and design; the brain organizes the material; and the mind experiences the beauty of the sunset. But what exactly is the mind, and has anyone ever seen the mind? Perhaps it is just a portal or the gateway for the infinite number of possibilities available for final causality. Remember when it comes to sex, the mind is supposedly the greatest aphrodisiac. That is because it is the mind that desires, seeks pleasure, and decides what is sexy and what is not. The mind turns us on! And it loves to fantasize.

Fantasy is a wonderful creation of the mind. The mind is the master of sexual fun. That is because when your thoughts are in a good place, your mind is in a good place; and sexual flirtation and attraction are more prevalent. So how do we get the mind sexually healthy? Remember this: thoughts are powerful things, and these powerful thoughts backed by a burning desire will become the material stuff of our dreams. There are no tricks and no fast tracks, but with determination and a little magic, we can create in material form whatever thoughts we want the mind to hold.

Everyone's mind is unique. No two minds think alike. That is because we all look out onto the world with our own perspective. Some of our perspective comes from nature and some by nurture. How you see the world is a direct reflection of your experiences, knowledge, desires, and pleasures. So what one mind holds as desirable may not be desirable in the mind of another person, and what brings pleasure to one person may not bring pleasure to another. To experience sexual health it is important that both partners share the same pleasures and desires.

As well as we create attraction, there are many ways to destroy it. How you look at the world and what energy you give off can destroy love. If you always have to be right, are always looking for perfection, and are critical of others, you will push love away. On the other hand, if you carry the victim mentality, inflict self-loathing, are angry, depressed, and lacking in self- confidence, love has nowhere to enter into your life. Excitement, joy, sensuality, and love all enhance sexuality. The magic of love is that when you send out loving messages, love comes back to you.

Now stop here for a moment. Sit back, close your eyes, and listen with all your senses. Picture yourself happy, playful, flirtatious, and friendly. This is the energy that causes people to respond to you positively. Everyone loves a flirt. You get compliments, smiles, and you feel sexy. You draw positive energy to you rather than being negative and repelling energy. Envision this within your mind and then get out and live it. The magic of love rests within you!

I know it is hard to be loving, playful, and happy when you are lonely. However, if you throw off positive energy, when the time is right, good things will come your way. Remember, you are what you think. If you are overly obsessed with finding love and having sex, or cynical about love and sex, you may be projecting negative energy that will keep you in a state of loneliness. Remember, if love is not in your life right now and you are truly open to finding love, it may not be the right time for love to come in. Your lover may not be ready to meet you, but destiny will bring your lover to you if you are open and ready when he or she arrives. Love will come if you will let it in.

As much as we think a perfect body, a smile, big breasts, or a strong jaw are sexually attractive, it's really the mind and that thing called chemistry that draw people together. Isn't it amazing that as we mature through life it is the mind that fuels desire and pleasures and not the pure physical act of sex? Our perception is what determines our reality and our reality is grounded in experiences, values, morals, and beliefs. The alchemists of the ancient world placed importance upon gaining knowledge and wisdom and knew that with age came experience, and with experience came the potential for wisdom.

Wisdom was seen as the most important thing a wise one could hand down to his or her prodigy. The alchemists knew that it took time and patience to turn lead into gold. It takes time (experience and patience) to turn the raw material of youthful lust into a mature and fulfilling love. The biggest detriment to a sensual and sexual life is fear. Fear is based on the ego's desire to control. It is the ego that pulls us back from falling in love. We hold back for fear of rejection and possible humiliation. In yoga, we are taught that there are three basic fears from which all other fears arise: the fear of not being accepted, the fear of not being loved, and the fear of dying. Of all the fears in life, the fear of not being loved ranks high on the list. Not being loved dovetails with rejection, and rejection is something the ego cannot handle.

Resentment, anger, disappointment, and pride all work to destroy any chance at finding and experiencing real love and sexual pleasure. We also become complacent and bored in our relationships, taking each other for granted. The excitement, the fantasy, the desire that was so prevalent in the mind in the beginning becomes a trap of routine chores and daily rituals. The passion, the excitement, the joy that once filled our thoughts has been dulled by time. Negativity, loneliness, and self-pity are not very attractive features. So what do we do to get the mind focused in the right direction? Have a little faith and believe in love.

A healthy mind is one that has a balanced and realistic outlook on life. It is not about trying to be positive and optimistic every waking moment of the day. That would be impossible. There will be up moments and there will be down moments. Balance means to walk the middle way — meaning that we let life flow and don't let emotionality sway us too far off balance. We stay centered with or without love in our life. Of all the treasures of evolution, the mind is the greatest because the mind can choose and direct the very existence of our life. The mind is free to choose.

To bring the mind into balance, we must become aware. Aware of what? Aware of the true nature of our being, including our desires and pleasures. And the wonderful paradox of awareness is that, as we become aware of our innermost being, things in our life begin to change. As events in our minds can be influenced by thoughts, so can events in our lives be influenced by the thoughts you hold in your mind. Resentment, anger, and fear hurt us and hurt others. So first, we need to reach inside our own mind and look at what thoughts, moods, perceptions, attitudes, and beliefs are preventing us from experiencing happiness and joy. When we truly look inside, the ego becomes transparent. We can literally pull back from ourselves and watch the ego play out its games. Awareness of this will stop the drama and games in our lives and bring to us a healthy and satisfying sensual and sexual life. If sexual desire begins in the mind, and if the mind is healthy and balanced, a healthy sex life will follow suit.

Meditation is the best way to clear the mind of negativity and plant into it the seeds that will grow healthy thoughts into physical realities. A quiet mind makes room for sensual thoughts. When we are relaxed and peaceful, the moment intensifies and our playful side has an opportunity to be revealed.

The mind is a fertile ground from which anything is possible. To get the mind sexy, we need to think sexy. But thinking sexy is a lot more than simply fantasying about a position, a person, or an act. A sexy mind is something that carries us through the day and manifests itself in the way we walk, talk, laugh, play, and interact with life. We see it in the bounce of a step, the wink of an eye, and in the seductive glance. What we think is what we become, so we need to think what we want to be to make it materialize.

This concept has a name. It is autosuggestion. Autosuggestion is self- suggestion. It means that all stimuli that we let enter the mind through self- suggestion will eventually manifest into physical reality. If we want something to manifest, we must have a clear and focused mind. The thoughts we put in our minds are what will appear in our life. It works like this: be very clear, about what you want, and then repeat over and over again in your mind the nature of your desire. However, these words and thoughts must be accompanied by a strong belief that what you desire will, in fact, materialize. You must have faith. Otherwise, the words and thoughts lack the vibration needed to bring the imagined into the tangible. This is not an easy task and will take a lot of self-discipline. For example, I know a woman who one week wants to meet a man and have a relationship. When it doesn't happen within the next week she says she never wants to meet anyone. She likes being alone. What does she want? If she cannot be perfectly clear and stay focused, how can the universe deliver?

However, before we can apply the power of autosuggestion we must put healthy loving thoughts into our minds. We must also be realistic about our desires. If you live in Kansas and desire falling in love with a Hollywood star, you may be living in a world of unreal expectations. If you truly want to meet someone beyond your reach, ask yourself honestly, what do I need to do to make this happen? Am I willing to move to Hollywood and take the steps to meet this person? Be honest.

What do you think of yourself? What do you tell yourself about yourself? Are you happy with your life as it is at the moment? If you say no and you want to make it better, remember it begins and ends with you. It has been said that when you are happy and not looking, love will find its way to your door. That is because you have total faith and have learned how to release your desires with complete belief into the universe. Whatever thoughts you release will come back to you. However, you must release them with faith and not obsess or get discouraged if what you desire does not come to you immediately. It is called contentment with what is in your life at the moment while being totally open to receiving what you desire most. If you obsess and get discouraged, the energy cannot manifest. Creation demands time, patience, and determination. Throughout my life, I have been able to manifest my desires. I have also drawn negative people and things into my life from obsessing and being discouraged. Negative energy only makes it take longer for positive energy to get into your life. Contentment is grounded in faith. It is a clear understanding that whatever is in your life or not in your life at this moment is for your own evolution. But how can that be? How can illness, loneliness, and emotional trauma be good for you? There is a message and something to learn. In the Great Dialogues of Plato, Plato tells us that in everything there is an element of good. We simply need to find it and focus on it, and then the lesson will be learned. Oftentimes we learn more from pain than from pleasure.

Two years ago exactly from the time of this writing (June 2010), I was diagnosed with cancer after being sick for nearly a year. I had to have a radical hysterectomy. Probably the scariest words to hear is your doctor tell you have cancer and we need to operate. The pain, the sickness, the trauma, and the fight back to health were a struggle. It was humbling and eye opening. I had struggled in my life with money, love, work, raising children, and educating myself but never had I really struggled with my health. This was beyond my control. For the first time in my life I experienced what it was like to not be able to get out of bed and "bull" my way through things. I learned humility, reverence, and respect for life and for my health. Nothing should be taken for granted. If you have your health you have everything. It's been two years, and so far I'm cancer-free. Anyone who has gone through cancer knows that in the back of your mind lurks the possibility that it can come back again. These thoughts, however, quickly spring back to a place of hope and appreciation. I have a different perspective on life. Out of every failure, problem, and tragedy will come an equivalent opportunity. You simply need to be open to the possibilities. If a love scorns you, another will come to take its place unless you allow the hurt, disappointment, and anger to rule your life.

Contentment does not mean that we simply accept what is and never reach out for more. It means we reach out with balanced energy, allowing the life force to flow to us rather than try to force it to us through negative and greedy means. A healthy mind begins with contentment, right here and right now, no matter what is in our lives at this very moment. Remember, everything is constantly changing; nothing is permanent. So to find contentment, we must be willing to flow with life rather than to resist and fight against it. The mind and our thoughts are just like the body. To create the desired results we must work at it. We must give the mind a "mental workout." Apply a little neuro-aerobics: diet, exercise, positive thoughts, relax, do a little meditation; and then repeat over and over, through the process of autosuggestion, your desires. Professional athletes employ the same techniques to win the game. Over and over, the athlete will practice strengthening the body and, at the same time, training the mind to focus on winning the game.

In general, we simply repeat through mental visualization our deepest desires. Whatever thoughts you hold in your mind will eventually materialize. Remember you cannot control other people, the weather, death, taxes, and many things in life. What you can control and influence is yourself. If you are sitting in (as we say in Maine) East Bum F--- and fantasizing about meeting and falling in love without a plan or a realistic view of your world, the chances are you are doomed. However, if you really want to meet and fall in love with someone, ask yourself, what you need to do to get there, and is it really what you want? Are you willing to do what it takes to make your dreams materialize? Remember, everything brings with it a price. Focus on what you can do and what you can control, do your very best and your dreams will come true.

However, there is one more thing you need to develop — a healthy and realistic self-image. But, you may think, I am unhappy and lonely; I am disappointed with my life. How can I get past this and have a healthy self- image when the media is constantly pitting us against perfection?

It begins with a realistic look at life. Hollywood and fashion magazines love to tell us what a sexy image is. For most of us, we could never quite measure up to those picture-perfect images. Most models are airbrushed, Photo shopped, touched up, professionally made up and styled to look perfect. However, you must remember, it is not the perfect sexual physical image that sells. That just gets a person's attention. Beyond the initial attraction, there must be the sexual allure to make things happen. That is why sex sells. It is not the image but the imagination behind the image, and that all takes place in the mind. Therefore, if you want your sex life to sizzle, the first thing you need to do is think good thoughts about yourself.

Let me share with you a secret. Most men and women are attracted to sex appeal over a contrived, sexy look. Next time you see a person who does not fit the perfect image but is getting lots of attention and having lots of fun, watch their body language. Take the time to feel and absorb their energy. Watch sex appeal in action. It all begins in the mind, because *life truly becomes what life does;* so think yourself sexy, and watch what happens. Flirt, play, have fun, and you will tap into your sexual and sensual self. Let go of the fear, because there is nothing to fear but fear itself.

And here is the great secret that, if applied, will manifest into your life whatever you desire. Whatever you make sacred, whatever you commit to, becomes the essence of your life. Most people live by the maxim that if it feels good just do it, and when the thrill is gone move onto something else. This doesn't mean you blindly commit to a person, place, or thing but rather; you commit to live your life to its greatest potential. This is the stuff that makes dreams come true. In a life without commitment, emotional neurosis happens. When we are focused and committed with a single pointed view, we can create anything we desire. It is all in the mind's eye. You are truly what you think!

In yoga, there are three mind states. The positive, which is optimistic; the negative, which looks at the worst; and the neutral, which sees both sides equally and offers up the best options. Every time we think positively, there is another part of the mind that thinks negatively. It becomes a vicious cycle that keeps the average person in a state of conflict and confusion. The neutral mind negotiates between the two and arrives at the best-case scenario. The neutral mind is not a given, it must be achieved through constant evaluation, contemplation, and inner quietude. It is from the neutral mind that our intuition springs forth. It represents balance, and a balanced state is a healthy mind. Sexual health begins in the mind. What you think is what you become. In the chapter *The Seven-Day Plan*, I will present you with a few mind exercises to get your *mojo workin'*.

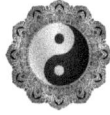

~ A successful life: to endure the betrayal of false lovers and false friends. ~

THE WAY OF THE HEART –
THE SPIRITUAL DISCIPLINE
OF LOVE AND SEX

The way of the heart in a spiritual sense is called sacred love. It is the journey of the heart toward the spiritual experience of love and erotic lovemaking. It asks, is love and erotic pleasure something we learn or is it something we experience by pure chance, if we are lucky? If love and erotic pleasure are to be learned, then the radiant force of sacred lovemaking requires knowledge, wisdom, and self-effort or a sense of self-discipline to perfect the art. The Eastern mystical paths of love and devotion, unlike the Western approach, require a sense of self-discipline. To experience the depth of eroticism requires a deep sense of intimacy, the intimacy that can be found only through the process of self-awareness. The ultimate goal of all mystical paths is to reach a state of total awareness so that the ordinary becomes the extraordinary, where the sacredness of bliss is experienced.

Most people see the problem with love as that of being loved rather than that of loving or of establishing within oneself the capacity to love. Hence, people think the problem is how to be loved or how to be lovable. They see the problem not as how to learn to love, but how to find the object to love and to receive love back.

In pursuit of finding the object of love, men seek to be powerful, successful, and strong, while women seek to be attractive and provocative. Cultivating good manners and being interesting and worldly are seen as attributes in the pursuit of love.

One of the major errors about the nature of love is the confusion between the initial "falling" in love, and the permanent state of being in love. When initially falling in love, two strangers begin to let down the walls between them and experience a moment of closeness or oneness that is exhilarating and exciting. It is, of life's experiences, the most intense and satisfying. If both people have been without love, isolated and lonely, it is even more intense. This intense intimacy is usually followed by sexual intimacy. However, this is not the intimacy of lasting love. As the two people become better acquainted, they begin to discover gaps of compatibility, disappointment, and boredom. Yet in the beginning, they believe that this infatuation with each other is proof of love. Often, however, it is simply the measure of their degree of loneliness and lack of self-knowledge and self- worth.

We believe that love is difficult to find and, yet, once we find the object of infatuation, we believe that it is an easy thing to maintain. However, statistics show that nothing fails as regularly as love. Since love is so important to us, it would seem that the only way to overcome the potential failure in the case of love is to examine the reasons for failure and to study the discipline for success.

The first step is to understand that love is something we learn and something we need to work at. If you wish to master something, you need to first master the theory and then master the practice. In any endeavor, we must commit to learning. It takes a great deal of knowledge and practice to become a master. In addition to the theory and the practice, to master an endeavor there must be commitment. To become the master, nothing in the world can be more important to the student than learning the process of a chosen endeavor.

Perhaps the problem lies in our focus on mastering, that which brings prestige and money over that which brings happiness and solace to the soul? In the East, the focus is called Bhakti yoga, the path of yoga that takes us to the "soul" of understanding the nature of sacred love and its expression through sacred sexuality.

Bhakti yoga is the path of conscious love that leads to harmonizing our personal relationships so that they serve the mutual spiritual process of discovery and transcendence. In the following pages, we will explore the various Eastern mystical approaches to Sacred Love and Erotic pleasures through the spiritual path of love.

The spiritual path of love makes the same claim as that made by ritual magic: *"If you follow a certain course of action with dedication and persistence, you will be led back to the roots of your own identity, you will learn the truth about yourself and the universe which you inhabit, and the nature of your existence will be transformed."*

Yoga is one of the Eastern approaches to discovering sacred love and erotic pleasures. There are six major branches of yoga. Bhakti yoga is one of the six major branches. Bhakti yoga is the path of self-transcending devotion. It means the all-embracing love of the divine, which is seen as being present in all of life. It may appear easy to open oneself to all encompassing devotion and love; however to experience Bhakti, the love must be pure and intense. The path requires emotional flexibility and the willingness to seek an open and truthful heart. Not an easy task.

Tantra yoga is a path of yoga that aligns itself with Bhakti. It is the path of self-transcendence through ritualism, which includes consecrated sexuality. Tantra is the way of action. All actions are undertaken with one purpose in mind: all actions are a means to an end. That end is the transformation of the individual to a new existence on all levels. There is no gap between the world and the divine; therefore, the divine can be found in ordinary life.

Tantra yoga is often misunderstood to be the practice of sexual rituals. It is considered to be the most esoteric of all the branches of yoga. Bhakti yoga is the way of the heart found through divine love and compassion, which is transformed into action through sacred sexuality; which is actually the path of Tantra. Tantra yoga is a path of rituals — sexual rituals being one of them. However, sex is only a small part. Tantra yoga is about realizing our creative potential, which is derived from the female energy of the universe or Shakti. The male energy Shiva unites with Shakti and creation is born. In reality, Bhakti and Tantra, like the other branches of yoga, are not strictly about adhering to Indian or Oriental philosophies. Both paths prescribe a way of life that is perfectly compatible with our modern Western culture.

An important expression of love is sexuality. The path of yoga promotes both sacred sex and celibacy. This, however, is often an area of conflict and frustration for many people. Sexuality and spirituality are not exclusive forms of self-expression. The sex drive in some Eastern schools of thought is to be used to enhance the energy of the soul and open us to a heightened level of spiritual awareness. These approaches are based upon the premise of sacred sexuality.

Celibacy, on the other hand, is also a powerful expression that can enhance the life force within us. However, celibacy does not necessarily mean abstaining from sex, as we shall see later in this book.

Bhakti yoga, although over 5000 years old is as relevant today as it was in ancient times. By inviting the sacred energy into our heart, we use our intimate relationships to actively transform our lives and align ourselves with the ideals of yoga; which is to yoke or bring into union the energy of the body, mind, and spirit through a self-imposed discipline that leads to inner and outer joy and harmony.

Bhakti is a Sanskrit (Indian) word for love. It means to participate and love through sacred sex, which is the most profound human form of participation. This love is seen as one of the devotional paths that lead to deity realization. It is the reconciliation of opposites or the male and female energies. We become one, not only with our beloved, but also with all that exists in the universe. The expression "love is blind," then, means that love makes no distinction, but extends out to everything and everyone.

When we talk of loving someone, we often speak of his or her charm, wit, looks, or style. This is the love of infatuation and not the true essence of love. True love cannot be quantified because it is about a person's true inner spiritual essence.

True love is the need to merge completely with another. It is ability to release the boundaries without losing the devotion, excitement, and desire to experience the greatest aspect of self and another through the experience of unconditional love. The Hindu scriptures refer to this as the union of the masculine energy (Shiva) and the feminine energy (Shakti). These two forces are the yin and the yang of the universe, as expressed through Buddhism and Taoism.

Shakti often appears as Shiva's wife. The two are seen in passionate and intimate embraces. This is because, in the Hindu religion, the body has always been considered an integral part of spirituality. Through the Hindu branch of yoga known as Tantra, one does not seek to control the desires of the body but aims at self-realization by engaging the body, the mind, and the soul. Enlightenment is found through intense sensual love in which the opposing forces of the universe (male and female) become one.

When Shiva (man) is portrayed in the sexual intimate embrace of his wife (Shakti), he is said to lose all sensation of what is within or without his being and experiences the sacred embrace of becoming one. This is the experience of complete union. As with the body-mind connected in an intimate embrace through intercourse, so it is experienced at the depth of the soul.

Our state of being (in the womb) prior to our initial realization of self is said to be one of pure love and bliss. Our need for love, passion, and devotion are said to be manifestations of our innate experience of this pure love and bliss. Bhakti yoga, along with Tantra yoga, makes use of our human emotions and experiences to awaken in each of us our true identity and return us to that initial state of pure love and bliss. Bhakti and Tantra take our love and bliss into the infinite possibilities of creation.

Bhakti yoga in the purest sense is the yoga path of devotion. The path seeks through dedication, commitment, discipline, and devotion to experience the Divine. In yoga, this means to find enlightenment or your inner spiritual essence. It is about seeking the truth within you. When you experience the truth of your pure essence, you experience the divine energy within and discover the unity of all. This is much like the path of the ancient alchemist who sought to find the Philosopher's Stone (the true essence of life) through a process of distillation. Although the craft of converting metals to precious substances was taught and practiced, the alchemist journey was really an allegory for discovering the divine energy within the entire universe.

Bhakti, like alchemy, requires devotion and discipline. To master the art of yoga or alchemy, one needs to devote his or her life to the search for the essence of life, which is unconditional, pure divine love. This quest for the pure essence of life has fascinated humankind since the emergence of human culture, which is believed to be as a result of rituals. Some anthropologists believe that rituals are the defining element that separated humans from other animals. Rituals define different cultures, and some rituals define us all as human beings. A smile, a kiss, a hug, a tear, and a celebration are universal. Rituals have always been used to search for the answers to life's mysteries. Love is one of life's greatest mysteries and is, after the basic needs of survival, the strongest human desire. Love has been the impetus for rituals of great creativity and rituals of great destruction.

The alchemist's works are based upon the search for the Philosopher's Stone, which is like much Bhakti yoga. Both contain within their context a message that may not be apparent on the surface. The Philosopher's Stone is not really a stone but rather a divine and earthly substance from which something of relatively worthless form is transformed into a precious substance. This substance is the essence of creation. Just like the search for the Philosopher's Stone — within the context of the Bible, the Holy Grail, and other such mystical and spiritual works — there are suggested allegorical stories that give birth to deep and mysterious secrets. Bhakti yoga is also one such work.

In the days of alchemy, the alchemist of the Middle Ages sought to transform the base metals of lead and iron into gold. It was believed that if one could take the basic properties and through a distillation process remove the impurities, the result would be of divine origin. In the alchemist's view everything — from sand and stone, to plants and people — had a physical body, a mind, and a soul. The art consisted of dissolving (distillation) the physical body and condensing it into the quintessence of life (the precious substance).

Although the mystical work continued to weave the quest for physical mastery into the quest for spiritual wisdom, it was the quest for the divine word of creation that predominated. It was believed that the true heavenly stone was, in fact, the word of the divine, and its purpose was to tinge the soul for salvation and eternal life. This divine word would lead one to the universal tincture (nectar) that would turn the ordinary into the extraordinary, but could only be found by those who followed the prescribed steps that would lead to the word of the divinity.

The alchemist's work emphasized transmutation of the spirit rather than the physical world. Man was presented as iron in unconverted *will* and purpose, and it was this unconverted *will* as well as the thoughts of earthly desire that must be transmuted into the purity of the divine.

It was believed that when transmutation was achieved the creature (humankind) and the creator would reunite and the soul would be free of vice, the heart would be dedicated to virtue, and one would experience the purity of unconditional love for all of creation.

The basic foundation of all things was seen as the spirit of divinity, and to discover the spiritual essence within was to be able to know all things. The highest form of unity was therefore revealed through the diversity of life, and this diversity through transmutation must return to the unity of creation. And so is it with the practice of Bhakti yoga, where the highest ideal of the souls of a man and a woman are to experience the diversity through unity and, thus, create the ecstasy of pure divine love through sacred sexuality.

To experience the purity of life, the ancient alchemist adepts placed great importance upon gaining knowledge and wisdom. Wisdom was believed to be the most important thing to attain in life. It was the quintessence of life. To turn the hard, unconverted lead to the purity of gold took time and patience and could only be achieved through devotion, dedication, knowledge, and discipline. This was the path of wisdom, which was considered the ultimate purpose of life. It is to realize the ultimate truth.

Let us define wisdom as a basic knowledge of universal truths, blended with values and meaning based upon an understanding that clarity is not always possible, and that much of life is unpredictable and uncertain. It is the ability to accept the fundamental truth of uncertainty in a state of peace and harmony that turns lead to gold.

In the Bhagavad-Gita (the new testament of Hinduism), it is taught that the purpose of yoga is to control the agitation of the wondering mind. This means to find clarity and accept uncertainty in a state of balance. We must always remember that we live in a material world, wherein, at every moment, our mind is subjected to agitation. We are always thinking that, by changing our circumstances, we will overcome agitation; and we believe that, when we reach a certain point in our lives, all mental agitation will disappear. But it is the nature of the material world that each new circumstance brings its own set of agitations. Therefore, the goal is to control the agitation of the mind no matter what the circumstances. This, yoga tells us, is done through devotion and renunciation of all desires.

In the Bhagavad-Gita, there are three basic types of yoga, Karma yoga, Jnana yoga and Bhakti yoga. The yoga system is like climbing a staircase, where we reach one level of practice, like Karma yoga — the path of cause and effect. We must practice at this level until we come to understand karma yoga and then master it before we can move to the next level. Otherwise, we remain in the karmic loop. Karma yoga is the path of discovering your life's work and purpose. It is the path of action. As long as we act out of egotism, we create desires, which blind us from our true identity. In blindness, we continue to repeat the never-ending cycle of karma — you reap what you sow. Karma yoga is the path that guides us to breaking the continual cycle of cause and effect and discovering our spiritual freedom through the discipline of work that is selfless and performed as a service to others.

In our modern-day Western society, our way of life demands that we make a living. Capitalism is not out of balance with Karma yoga. If the work is performed for the purpose of sharing, in balance and harmony with universal values, then we are performing that which will bring the greatest good. Prosperity is seen as good, as prosperity allows one to take care of and share with others. Finding purpose and meaning through karma yoga we move onto Jnana yoga.

Jnana yoga is the path of discernment and wisdom. As we grow and mature, we gain wisdom. This wisdom helps us to discern between what is unreal and what brings true happiness. We see the material world for what it really is and learn to detach from things that bind us to the never-ending cycle of negative karma. This leads us to Bhakti yoga.

Bhakti yoga, as stated before, is the path of self-transcending devotion. Although in its ultimate sense, Bhakti is about discovering the divine essence of the Godhead and through total devotion a renunciation of the material world, its application in the modern Western world can be that of spiritual love and union between man and woman, human to human, and all that exists.

The whole process of the yoga system is to purify oneself. Through purification (transmutation), one realizes true identity. It is the realization that "I am pure spirit — I am not the matter of the body." In the material world, we are constantly identifying with matter. The system of yoga teaches us to stop identifying with matter, find our true inner essence, which is pure spirit, and then incorporate that energy into our material lives. Bhakti yoga is about transcending the sensual boundaries of the physical world and learning to love from a place of devotion and pureness, which is the essence of the soul. Sex ceases to be physical gratification and becomes a sacred ritualistic connection of body, mind, and soul.

When the yogi engages with sincere effort in attaining the purity of self, free of all contaminates, it is said he or she has reached perfection. All yoga culminates in Bhakti yoga because Bhakti yoga is the rendering of devotional services through pure and unconditional love. Bhakti yoga is the ultimate goal or true path to eternal good fortune. Like alchemy, it is about the transformation of matter into pure essence.

To reach and practice Bhakti yoga is said to be the final link in the chain of higher consciousness, for Bhakti surpasses all other systems to where we attain the ultimate goal of yoga, which is unconditional pure love.

There is a prescribed set of steps in the study of yoga, which, if followed with dedication and persistence, will lead us back to the roots of our identity. One of the first steps to experiencing sacred love and erotic pleasures is to practice the laws of Abstention (Yamas) and the laws of Observance (Niyamas). We must learn to abstain from certain things and to observe certain things if we are to achieve the self-awareness necessary to experience the pureness of sacred love and erotic pleasures.

When we look carefully at nature, we see that nature unfolds rhythmically and harmoniously in relationship to all that exists. This rhythmic and harmonious enfoldment is what creates the cosmic consciousness of balance and harmony.

The practice of celibacy is one of the abstentions taught through yoga. It is one of the most misunderstood concepts. In the Western world, we believe celibacy to be abstention from all sexual activity. Although there are adepts who practice celibacy in the truest sense — it really means to control the sense organs. According to Hindu tradition, celibacy is practiced for the first few years of life, while the individual is a student. The next phase is that of the householder where a man and woman come together to form a family. The third phase of a person's life is a regaining of the control over the sense organs, and the final stage is a return to total celibacy as one finishes one's life with a total spiritual focus.

The Hindu holy text makes it very clear that procreation is a sacred sacrifice and a sacred ritual. The holy text states that the path of the householder is the best path for the average person. The process of procreation is seen as the realization that, through sacred sex, souls take on earthly birth.

The Gita (ancient text) points out that to be obsessed over objects of desire is to be attached. Attachment and desire create cravings, and cravings cause the mind to become scattered. The main purpose of celibacy is to control the senses (scattered mind) and preserve energy so one can obtain spiritual enlightenment.

According to the Gita, there are three important points regarding sexuality:

• The opposite sex should be held in high regard.
• Sexuality should be considered noble and as a means for bringing souls into the world.
• Nothing scatters the body-mind more than sexual cravings.

Therefore, in order to have balance in your life, when you meditate, meditate, when you eat, eat, and when you make love, make love. Therefore, *celibacy* means to do all things with gentleness and love, remain unattached, and allow the experience to unfold.

Verbal celibacy means to control your words regarding sexual expressions and overtones. This means we should always seek to express ourselves sexually with high regard and respect for the process of making love.

Practicing celibacy in thought and in speech makes it easy to practice physical celibacy. Physical celibacy can mean to abstain from sex entirely. However, the householder's approach to physical celibacy means to practice sex without attachment by controlling the sexual senses so that sex is performed in a noble and sacred manner. Ecstasy is a great experience in life, and sacred sex gives us an opportunity to experience the ecstasy of spiritual sex by controlling the attachment of the sex senses. It is more about the experience than the goal of orgasm.

To experience sex in a noble and spiritual manner is to taste the outer fringe of bliss. For most humans, making love is the closest experience they will ever get to experience the magnitude of life: the process of creation. If two people are really loving, touching, and giving. then the soul will experience the process and respond. People who have truly loved from the soul will understand the difference between sacred sex and non-sacred sex.

Loving is a process whereby we have the opportunity to touch another's soul. The joy and bliss a soul feels when he or she is moving into the ecstasy of sacred sex is beyond the physical plane. However, it is through the physical experience of sacred sex that the two souls truly connect.

Lovemaking is a way to direct great amounts of spiritual and loving energy to another soul. Only if you direct that energy with great love and respect will you receive the same force of energy in return. This is sacred sex and what it means to make love in a celibate manner.

Like the laws of yoga, love requires us to follow observances and abstinences if we are to experience the true nature of enduring sacred love. To realize the true nature of love, you must come to understand the unification of the two opposing forces of the universe: matter and spirit. The coming together of opposites brings the female and male energy into perfect union. This union is made manifest through our experiences; and through our experiences, we gain knowledge. This knowledge leads us to an understanding of the truth, which must be lived and experienced.

Nonviolence, another abstention, is an absolute requisite for the experience of love. This means we should always strive to act, think, and speak in a loving and gentle manner. If we cannot act, think, and speak without abuse and violence, then we should move away from the situation in peace and harmony. The dignity of your being is the dignity of your soul. True love would never tolerate abuse. Ask yourself who you are being in relationship to the object of your love. If you are being a loving and peaceful soul, then you are experiencing spiritual enlightenment; but if you are being angry, harsh, and violent, then you are compromising the dignity of your being and your soul.

Trust and respect are essential if one is to experience the nature of true love. Once trust is broken, a relationship suffers the loss of friendship, which is a deep and important part of any loving relationship. To understand truth you must search your own mind, speech, and actions to determine that, in fact, you are acting in accord with the truth. If one truly desires to love, then untruthfulness cannot exist because untruthfulness is the complete opposite of openness, which is how a relationship grows in strength. There must also be within you no intention to inflict harm. Truth must be unified in body, mind, and speech so that all our experiences and expressions are harmonious. This creates a steady body-mind, and a steady body-mind leads one down the path of wisdom. In wisdom, you will realize that you may be used by the world and hurt by others, but if you are truthful within yourself, you will always find solace and peace.

Non-stealing is another abstinence connected with love. Most people think of stealing as taking something from someone. This is also true regarding the abstinence of non-stealing, however, when referring to love, it means that we should not seek to steal another's pride, dignity, happiness, moments of glory, or mental values. We also should not deceive another person or force him or her into any situations that steal away their sense of self.

To abstain really means to control the senses towards uplifting of the soul. In many ancient texts such as *Tantra* and the *Kama Sutra*, lovemaking is a process whereby we learn through control of the senses to experience more than simply the carnal act of sex. Sexuality becomes the touching of another in such a way as to enlighten the soul. If one is truly connecting with another person, then the soul recognizes the connection and love is made at the soul level. So *abstaining* (celibacy) means to control and direct positive energy towards another in such a way that great physical and mental love is experienced. *Celibacy* means to abstain from purely physical or sensory pleasures and, instead, seek to find fulfillment and spiritual pleasure through the sharing of intimate energy with another.

Greed, another abstention, by its very nature can be devastating to a relationship. When greed is present, the sense organs are out of control. The thought process is not on how to connect with another but rather how to get what one wants in the moment. It is about immediate gratification. When we become attached to the objects of our desire, craving for pleasure and gratification intensify and can cause a person to commit violence against another and/or against him- or herself. We need to guard against greed because, once greed takes hold, we begin to reach out and want to possess others. Once we begin to feel the possession, we immediately begin to feel the fear of losing, and the body-mind becomes scattered with jealously. The agitated mind then loses its focus and the life force of love becomes scattered.

The purpose of the abstinences is to bring peace, tranquility, and serenity to your mind. Seek out wise ways to bring solace to the mind and the body will respond accordingly. Only if we can learn to balance our subconscious energies do we truly experience the bliss of love and devotion. Through the practice of Bhakti yoga (the yoga of devotion), you can take your conscious mind into your subconscious mind and produce within yourself gentleness and happiness, which are the prerequisites for finding true love.

As well as we must abstain from certain things, we must also learn to observe. To observe means to notice something and to pay special attention to it. True love demands that we notice the nuances of love and pay special attention to its ebb and flow. Observing, we learn to direct our energy in such a way that we pull the cosmic energy of unconditional love into our being. Yoga teaches that we must follow the five observances of purity, contentment, austerity, study, and attunement to a higher power if we are to experience the pureness of love.

Purity means that we think, act, and speak in such a way as to bring truthfulness and openness to our relationships. By drawing from our heart, we vow to evoke loving thoughts that bring peace and serenity to our relationships. Through our speech, we lift the energy of love from the heart area to our vocal chords where we express ourselves with words of love and kindness. *Physical purity* means that we act only in ways that are in accord with the nature of true love, which is compassion. We strive to love another through physical gestures that are warm and loving.

Contentment is considered the most vital of the observances, as it leads one to accepting rather than expecting. It means we should be accepting of what is in our life at this very moment and not expect more. Never be disappointed with your life, but reach out with quietude to find balance and serenity. This brings contentment, and contentment opens the door to lasting and real love.

Contentment also means that we should always be prepared to part with anything we do not need. Love is whimsical, and it comes and goes as it pleases. We should always be prepared to let it come when it will and let it go when it must. Love is established in abundance, which means as it departs it will come again as long as we don't become cynical and afraid.

Contentment further means that we should be content even when that which is taken from us hurts. That which we need more dearly at this time in our lives will replace it. Sometimes love must leave to make room for growth and evolution.

Physical contentment works with mental contentment in that we should seek to release ourselves from body language that manifests from thoughts, which might show emotional hurt and insults. When one is not content in body-mind, greed and obsession take over. Greed and obsession are sure to kill love. But if one can learn to be content and remove desires and cravings, one acquires everything and finds the true nature of love.

Austerity, another observance, is the power to withstand discomforts and not to have what you desire without losing the sense of self. Not having love in your life is one of the most difficult situations for most people. Most everyone wants to have love and a partner to share the wonders of life. Loneliness is a difficult state to accept and, yet, if you can find contentment in the austere world of aloneness, you open yourself up to finding a love that is real, lasting, and not based upon a craving, desire, or need.

Austerity means that we need to undergo hardships in order to attain happiness. Unless we can experience the nature of loneliness, how can we learn to truly appreciate companionship, friendship, and love? However, we need to be careful here. If we seek to fill the void of loneliness from a place of despair, we will end up only more alone and disappointed. To be alone and be happy and content opens the door to finding a healthy and balanced relationship.

If you are happy and content in your life, you will only draw into your life that which supports and enhances this state of balance and happiness. If you are discontent and lonely, you will draw into your life that which enhances the loneliness and discontentment. Therefore, in the austerity of life, you have an opportunity to discover your own inner balance through self-discipline and self-love, and in this state of being you open yourself up to finding a healthy and lasting love.

If you are living in austerity because of anger and stubbornness, you will become a dull and angry person.

If your sense of austerity comes from a cold and misguided place, then you are living within a false sense of control. Neither passion, anger, nor dullness will endure. Agitation, fear, and resentment will move in to take contentment's place. However, if your austerity is grounded in calmness your body-mind will be pure, serene, and open to everlasting happiness and thus contentment.

Yoga teaches that we should be moderate in all our activities and not exhaust ourselves with worry. When we stop clinging to desires, we free the energy of the body-mind to move. We move with grace and ease. And this will attract to us exactly what we need in our lives at this very moment for our own evolution.

This brings us to self-study, another observance. The use of mystical techniques and mystical texts leads to self-realization as well as an understanding of the fullness of life. In the study of self and love such texts as the *Kama Sutra* and *Tantra* should be studied, memorized, and applied through thoughts, words, and actions. We should also study spiritual scriptures and question the nature of things. As we learn more about the nature of life, so we learn more about the nature of ourselves. This leads one to understand the unity in all things, which, of course, includes human nature and the experience of love.

Physical self-study is essential in the pursuit of sacred love. How one carries oneself is an attractive feature and an indicator of the sensual and sexual nature of one's being. How we walk, dress, and adorn ourselves are symbols of our availability.

With affection, intimacy, and sex, the body must cooperate. Therefore, when you are making love, make love, and when you are being affectionate, be affectionate. Always be present and aware in body and mind. This is all part of self-study.

Diet and exercise, as well as rest, cleanliness, and proper posture, are manifestations of our awareness of self, both inside and outside. As you study yourself, you decide what type of a being you wish to be. This is true when it comes to sex and love. Great lovers totally understand the importance of awareness. It is what sets apart mere sex from that of intense lovemaking. means to move from the inquisitive exploration of the inner self to a revelation of the entire self — unified, balanced and content.

The fifth, and last, observance is an attunement to *Ishvar,* which is interpreted to mean an absolute and total dedication of all your actions toward your chosen higher power in life. This means that we strive to experience the unconditional love that is necessary to live a spiritual life.

From this center of divine love, sacred love will be found, and it will overflow into all area of our lives.

Attunement to *Ishvar* brings us to our center. Centering means to move toward the discovery of beauty and life's meaning as the sole purpose of being, rather than for the purpose of obtaining something. This final observance is the apex of all the other laws of love. Without the attainment of devotion and spiritual realization, it is impossible to dedicate your actions and the fruits of your actions away from cravings and desires and toward the experience of a sacred sense of love. Sacred love is pure, simple, and balanced. It has no agenda. It is simply the essence of pure love. When two souls come together from this perspective, devotional love and pure erotic pleasures are exchanged.

According to the *Kama Sutra*, the ancient Indian text, which is the guide to pleasures and sexual techniques, there are three aims in one's life and three phases of development. The three aims are virtue, prosperity, and love; and neither one should be more important than the other. All three must be lived out in balance and harmony.

The first phase of life is childhood, which ends at about sixteen. Up until this time, the child is to remain celibate and devote time to study and acquiring knowledge. The second phase is that of the lover and household keeper.

This means the pursuit of a relationship, which, of course, includes love and sex. The third phase is a return to celibacy. However, in the second phase, one should also be dedicated to acquiring wealth, as wealth or prosperity is the vehicle that allows one to give, allows a society to prosper, and provides for the means in the final years to contemplate life quietly with the ability to impart and share wisdom.

The second phase of life or the adult phase is a very complex stage. The pursuit of wealth often falls prejudice to the balancing act of love and relationships. Balancing time between lovemaking and building wealth with a sense of virtue, as the *Kama Sutra* tells us, is what it means to live a healthy and balanced adult life.

Love and sex are fundamental to any healthy relationship. Likewise, trust and respect must be present. The problem is that we often confuse love for lust, sex for self-gratification, and trust and respect for pride and ego.

Prosperity allows the individual to seek all three of the aims in life. For according to the *Kama Sutra*, there is no virtue in poverty. Poverty is seen as an obstacle to pleasure, ethics, and virtue. Morality is a luxury very poor people can rarely afford.

Ethics satisfies the conscience, love satisfies the mind, and spiritual enlightenment brings peace to the soul. Without food, clothes, and shelter the body becomes weak and dies. Without erotic and playful gestures, the mind becomes restless and dissatisfied. Without virtue (ethics), the conscience goes astray and without spirituality, the soul loses its integrity.

This is why the *Artha-shastra* (ancient Hindu treatise) teaches that, even when one is on the spiritual path, it is necessary to earn money and enjoy love and sex. The refinement of the arts and love can be experienced only in a prosperous society. This is why it is important to seek prosperity. However, the *Artha Shastra* and the *Kama Sutra* make it very clear that ethics, virtue, and non-attachment must also be observed.

Seeking money and pleasure, without considering the spiritual path of ethics and virtues, is materialistic and senseless. When people are attracted only to money and pleasure without virtue; greed, anger, deceit, and pride play powerful roles in destroying the beauty of a loving relationship.

However, without satisfaction of a material kind, it is difficult to follow the spiritual path. Just as the soul needs spiritual enlightenment, the body needs food, water, shelter, sex, and health, and the mind needs love and caring. Without material well-being and sexuality, life would cease to exist.

So, just as virtue and prosperity are essential to a civilized society, so is sexuality. Eroticism, like money and virtue, is an aid to the realization of spirituality, if approached from a virtuous point of view. To fulfill material well-being, sex, and virtue means to experience contentment and happiness. The quality of one's life is measured by the degree of happiness we experience. If something is lacking, such as our basic needs, dissatisfaction may lead to unhappiness. Happiness is therefore derived from our *relationship* to or with things and not our *attachment* to things. This is the practice of non-attachment.

Non-attachment means that we stop identifying with our needs, our likes and dislikes, and instead recognizes that we do have our needs, likes, and dislikes, and it is good to satisfy these without allowing them to have absolute hold over our happiness and contentment.

Most people find life to be difficult because they are locked into fear and the possession of things. Reaching out and attaching to things, the mind becomes fearful of losing them and easily becomes agitated. An agitated mind scatters your energy and creates jealousy and envy. This causes self to cling even harder to the object (person) of desire, draining the relationship.

The key word is *detachment*. It is not a detachment from things but from our reaction to things. It means to stand outside of everything and observe life as it unfolds in the moment. In the moment is the only reality. If what you have in the moment is good, then embrace it and enjoy it for what it is, but be prepared to release it should there be the next order of things. It means to experience "imperturbability," which means to not be perturbed (agitated) by what presents itself in your life or what leaves your life.

If you do not like what is in your life at this moment or you desire to have something else in your life at this moment, sit quietly in a state of contentment knowing that life is dynamic and ever-changing and always open to the infinite possibilities of the universe. In other words, in our quietude and contentment we find the stability and balance necessary to see things as merely backdrops to our lives. Things can come or go; it matters not, for no matter what, we still remain in a state of balance and contentment. We become the witnessing consciousness of our lives.

The very nature of creation is ever-changing form and abundance. From quiet balanced energy we gather the strength and clarity that is necessary to create whatever we desire. Desire is good for it is the motivation behind creation. However, attachment to the results without the flexibility to change creates a state of polarization and everything grinds to a halt. Nothing happens in a state of stagnation. Therefore, to free the self from attachment to results is to detach and enjoy without losing the passionate experience of creative desire. And here is the difference — creative desire is powerful where craving desires are destructive.

Non-attachment is the ability to let go of whatever must leave your life at this time and to not bemoan over what is not in your life at this time. Both leaving and not having are replaced by what is needed at this time in your life. When you become unattached to what flows in and out of your life there will always be balance and contentment and great opportunities will be revealed. In relationships, we experience this same kind of balancing act. We need to respect our own needs and wants and, at the same time, be able to step back from them and allow the boundaries to dissolve so we can unite with another. If we simply merge with another because of insecurities and discontentment, we risk becoming attached and losing ourselves in the relationship, which spells disaster.

We want our freedom and, at the same time, we want to unite with another and experience commitment and stability. We want belonging and love. However, to surrender to a relationship involves the giving up of something. To have one thing, we must be willing to let go of another. This is the contradiction — the polarization that has the potential to bring a relationship to a standstill. We want closeness and, yet, desire our separateness. It is a dilemma and the contradiction of relationships.

The conflict that arises from our attached cravings and desires is the root of suffering. Buddhism teaches that all suffering results from our inability to face the true nature of things, which is ever-changing. We cling to the false notions of life. We cling to things believing they are permanent when, in fact, they are temporary; just like all of life. To end this suffering is to let go and simply flow with life. It is when we resist and cling that we get hurt.

Non-attachment is to find contentment in your life, even if what you desire is not present. At the same time, you should reach out with quietude toward that which you desire. Never be disappointed if what you desire does not come into your life, not overly elated if more than what you expect comes into your life. Stay balanced.

If you have not received that which you truly desire, it simply means you have not earned it yet. There may be more work you need to do or the time is not right. However, in quietude and faith one realizes the true nature of self — which is creation — and from this creative principle, each one of us has the power to create and achieve whatever we desire. But you must believe it to be true with absolute faith.

Contentment is the root of happiness because, in a state of contentment, the body-mind is free of all agitation and stress. This energy permeates out and manifest into the world. This manifestation is what you become and is the very energy force that will draw to you that which you truly desire.

A person not content will spend all of his or her energy trying to obtain objects for enjoyment. This brings possessiveness and disappointment, for objects never bring contentment. This, of course, leads to fear and clinging, which is the vicious circle of attachment and discontentment.

Remember this significant point regarding your desire to find sacred love and erotic pleasures: When you reach out into the world with quietude, balance, contentment, and non-attachment, you create an energy that draws to itself the kind of love and pleasure that every human being desires.

Bhakti, as well as meaning love, also means to participate. Love is considered the most profound participation of which we are capable of experiencing. It means to touch the very essence of another person. This can be confusing in the Western culture as we often attribute love to the way a person looks or acts. However, if we truly love, it is the indefinable and unqualified essence of the person with which we connect; that is the essence of love. Sacred love is the desire of the soul to merge completely with another soul. It is the realization that, at the highest level, we are all connected.

Bhakti yoga makes use of the personal feelings of compassion, devotion, empathy, respect, and honesty as the elements of true love. It is about awakening to our true identity, which is pure love and bliss, then taking that love-bliss, and extending it out into everything and everyone in the universe. The problem is that our egos and sense of self-gratification get in the way.

The truth is that we are all quite self-centered and that we spend a lot of time trying to control others. We enter into relationships to end loneliness, find security, have a family, end depression, and for ego gratification. All of these reasons are ways of seeking to control from a state of fear. None of these reasons brings happiness and love. This was the ultimate quest of the alchemist, using the allegory of turning lead to gold as a hidden message of how to turn the lead of our ego and its attachment to the material world, into the pure essence of life (gold) which, in turn, is to fully surrender and experience the pure and ultimate essence of love.

To transcend the attachment and control of the ego is to find spiritual love. It is an awareness of the sacredness and blessedness of connecting with another at the soul level. It is about giving love, not receiving love back, but because love must be given to become complete and fulfilled.

Spiritually, our natural state is that of pure unconditional love and bliss. Our desire is to create that same state of love and bliss through the relationship or merging with another human being. Bhakti yoga teaches us to use human emotions in a positive way to rediscover the original love bliss experience.

A love relationship is a powerful dance of polarity. As we attempt to merge with another person, we experience seduction, eroticism, and delight and sometimes fighting, resistance, and combative energy. A love relationship can be energizing or exhausting.

When we find ourselves attracted to another person, the dance begins. At first, we desire to break out of our separateness and merge with another in a way that stretches beyond all our boundaries. Then, we begin to experience the fear of giving up too much and losing ourselves. The dance of love always involves moving between the coming together and the moving apart. It is not an easy dance to master.

Many couples lose the coming together and moving apart rhythm and wind up in opposing positions, attacking and withdrawing. How to keep from falling out of rhythm and avoid polarity is found in a set of prescribed steps for finding sacred love.

The secret to finding sacred love is not about satisfying the body-mind, but about establishing yourself in spiritual awareness. This opens the doorway to a deeper and more meaningful relationship. When the connection between two people is based upon spiritual balance and insight, the souls connect, honesty exists, and each individual respects and honors the nuances of the other. There is a deeper realization that we are all interconnected and that to find one's soul mate means transcending beyond the focus on our earthly needs and seeking a deeper meaning and understanding of what it means to have the human experience of unconditional love.

Sacred love is a process whereby we bring forth the illumination of another soul, moving past the physical plane and into the realm of pure joy and bliss. People who have truly loved will understand that nothing in the universe can touch us so deeply as connecting with the soul of another person. When the spiritual element is missing in a relationship, emptiness and disappointment is sure to follow. To find a soul mate there must be a willingness to surrender to the process of your own spiritual inner work. Carefully examine the following prescribed steps, which will take you through the process of enlightenment and open you up to finding a love relationship beyond anything you have ever known.

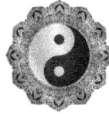

~ A successful life: to both cry and laugh with deep emotion. ~

THE PRESCRIBED STEPS

COMPATIBILITY – STEP ONE

I f you have chemistry without compatibility, you have lust; and if you have compatibility without chemistry, you have friendship. The union of chemistry and compatibility can bring us into a place of deep emotional experience.

Compatibility, by definition, means to get along or to go well together. There is an intimacy of sorts, but in its purest sense, it lacks passion and commitment and is what makes for enduring friendships.

When it comes to the intimate, passionate union between a man and a woman, compatibility is often overlooked. Instead, the couples are so focused on the sex and the passion that they neglect the need to establish the intimacy of a shared approach to the basics of life. This means that what we eat, how and when we sleep, and how we choose to keep our homes (tidy or scattered) can have adverse effects on a relationship. Sexual desires and financial compatibility are essential to the health of a relationship. Sex and money are two factors that can make or break a relationship. Most fights are of a sexual or financial nature.

Enjoying the same foods, having similar sleeping patterns, liking the same recreational activities, and having the same level of sexual drive are all factors that need to be considered before entering into a relationship. Religious affiliations and political views, as well as spending and saving habits, are elements of compatibility. Without an examination of each other's lifestyle habits and preferences, problems are sure to surface.

If compatibility is such an important part of a relationship, why do we give it minor importance? Probably because the sexual urges of romantic love, where passion is the overriding factor, clouds our ability to be reasonable and logical. Chemistry may be at fault and, yet, in the pure nature of things, it is chemistry and not compatibility that ensures the survival of the species. Nature has designed its mortality in such a way that the fires of passion lead to procreation without thought or concern with what comes afterwards. This, of course, works in all species of plants and animals accept for humans, some other mammals, and a few other species that need pair bonding, commitment, and continuation for survival. Humans mate for pleasurable reasons and not necessarily for reason of procreation.

Lifestyle and personal choices must be examined in the context of a committed relationship. When mixed with chemistry the relationship takes on an exciting and deeply intimate level. Both partners share in the enjoyment of a compatible life. They enjoy each other, being together, and sharing common interest. They enjoy sleeping together, eating together, and playing together, which are essential elements of a balanced and healthy relationship.

The key factor in attachment or bonding is a sense of security and comfort that is part of being with a favored person. When this is mixed with intimacy, affection, and sex, we have what can be termed a consummate love. The *Kama Sutra* states that if one wants to succeed in love, incompatibilities should be considered before making love.

INTIMACY – STEP TWO

Intimacy is the ability to fuse yourself with another person without fear of losing yourself — meaning that, until one has established a true sense of self, it is nearly impossible to fuse with another sexually or any other way. Unsure of our identity, we shy away from intimate relationships. As we gain a greater sense of identity, we begin to seek the true intimacy of love.

Many people make the mistake of thinking that they will find their identity in another. This is often the problem in young adult relationships. These relationships remain shallow, and the individual ends up feeling isolated and alone.

Intimacy is a feeling that promotes closeness and connectedness. This is the most crucial part of a loving relationship because it provides the backdrop for confidentiality. Without having our mate as our confident, we suffer isolation. Intimacy is the ability to open oneself up completely without fear. It means to find acceptance in another through the disclosure of the most intimate details of our lives. To do this with a passionate and loving mate can take the sexual experience to heightened portions.

Sharing your innermost thoughts, fantasies, and dreams is a wonderful experienced. Intimacy comes when we clearly have a strong identification with ourselves and have dropped the fears and insecurities. With a strong identification and a true sense of self-love and acceptance, we are free to drop the barriers and experience the depth of intimacy. This is one of the beginning steps to finding sacred love and erotic pleasures.

AFFECTION – STEP THREE

B y definition, *affection* means fond and tender feelings. To be affectionate means to display those tender and loving feelings. This is usually done through hugging, kissing, and caressing. Of course, we can do things like cook a nice meal or bring flowers to show affection.

Without the tenderness and loving expression of affection between two people, a relationship loses intimacy. When affection is lost, a relationship falls into what is known as empty love. An empty-love relationship is one where there is commitment without passion or intimacy. The relationship becomes stagnated, whereby mutual involvement and attraction are lost.

Physical affection is necessary for happiness and growth. Without touching and fondling, infants die and adults slip into depression and anxiety. We all need to be touched and hugged in a loving and affectionate manner. Love is not necessarily sex, although sensual gratification in the form of touching and affectionate gestures is a part of loving. Affection is a form of loving and, of course, may lead to sex.

Our social mores often prohibit public displays of affection. Some people even look upon holding hands as a taboo. However, when you touch someone, you experience his or her realness and his or her warmth, or the lack thereof. Touch is pleasurable and displays of affection usually include touching.

Some people do not like to be touched and will pull away from another's advances. This is their right and must be respected. However, love is physical and expressive and, by its very nature, demands physical affection.

If affection is the display of fond and loving feelings, then affection sparks the intimate emotions of the mind into play through the physical expression of the body. Affection is truly a body-mind experience where we merge together in a spirit of love the deep sensation of giving. In love's greatest depth, it is about the need to give from your heart and your soul without fear. When fear and hidden agendas disappear, one has the opportunity to express and experience the depth of affection.

COMMUNICATION – STEP FOUR

The single, biggest problem we face as human beings is communication. Everything in life involves some form of communication. However, it is miscommunication, with all its nuances, that causes all our problems. The major reasons most relationships fail is a lack of honest and open communication. This takes trust, respect, and caring. Communication is an expression of love, both verbally and non-verbally.

Relationships are work. They demand that we constantly work at understanding and growing with another, within the relationship and within ourselves. To communicate with another in an effective manner requires we take the time to listen. To listen means to listen not only to words but also to how something is being said, and to the manner in which it is said. We must learn to pay attention to the subtleties of body language.

Why is communication such a major problem in relationships? Because we fear rejection and lack the necessary skills to effectively discuss our fears and disappointments. It is very difficult for us to communicate our needs and desires to another. We call this conflict, and conflict resolution often ends in either fighting or taking flight (running away) from the situation.

To effectively communicate within a relationship, both parties must be committed to the process. The process of communication demands honesty, openness, and the willingness to compromise, see the other's point of view, and work towards harmony and mutual satisfaction. The key word is commitment to making the relationship work based upon mutual desire.

SEX – STEP FIVE

Your sexuality and your orientation define you. Long before human consciousness develops, nestled in the womb, we are either a male or a female, or in other words a sexual being. From conception, the nature of our lives is determined. We are and will always be a sexual being. In mystical terms, we are either male in search of our female half or female in search of our male half. Birth and the human development of our sexuality assist us in finding our other half and becoming complete.

Our ultimate desire in life is love and acceptance. Everything we do in our lives is merely an attempt to reach a state of unconditional love and unconditional acceptance. Sex is a major factor in the drive and desire to achieve this state of being. Although there is a physical drive fueled by hormones and peptides, as humans, it is the ultimate connection of love and acceptance that we desire. Sex provides the connection.

The most basic element of the human sexual response is for procreation. It is through sex that the species ensures survival. Nature has endowed the universe with sensual aids to ensure the procreation of nature. However, the human element is far more complex. We have feelings, emotions, expectations, and desires. Beyond the physical pleasure, human sexuality serves as an important reinforcement of pair-bonding and an emotional connection between two individuals. This is what separates us from the rest of the animal kingdom.

Who would deny that sex is an important element in a happy and healthy relationship? However when issues and problems develop in a relationship, sex is often the first thing to go. Without sexual contact couples tend to drift apart, given there are no health issues and the couple is still able to actively pursue sex.

Probably the most difficult part of our sexual lives is the familiarity that develops in long-term relationships. The excitement of the newness and exploration of each other gives way to routine sex. The demands of work, family, and social commitments can interfere in the time we give to keeping the sexual fires burning. Not to mention the fact that, in time, we get to know the everyday existence of each other, and the intrigue and desire give way to boredom.

Researchers at Duke University conducted a study on sexual activity beginning with couples in their twenties through couples in their sixties. They concluded that couples in their twenties, on average, have sex ten or more times per month, and then it drops to about three times per month in the sixties. The decline however has many factors, which include duration of the relationship, mental outlook, and declining health.

As early as our thirties, we start to experience hormonal changes. As the body begins to decline, subtle changes in our libido occur. However, like all things in nature the outcome is determined by many factors. If we abuse our bodies with poor diet, alcohol, drugs, and sedentary lifestyles, there is a good chance that our sex lives will suffer.

Since sex is such an important part of a healthy and happy relationship, it is vitally important that we take care of our health and learn to keep our erotic desires strong. Without health and eroticism, the drive of sex diminishes. Given that sex is such an important part of our health and our lives, it seems vitally important that we look at not only the sexual act but also how eroticism and desire can enhance our lives.

Love is not the result of sexual satisfaction. However, sexual happiness can lead to love and commitment. Sexual happiness and compatibility usually lead to continuation of the relationship, and although this is no guarantee that the relationship will continue, it is a factor regarding commitment.

What appears to be frigidity in women and impotence in men, given no health factors or deep psychological factors, is oftentimes a lack of desire or attraction for one's partner. When sexual attraction disappears, it is difficult to initiate sex. As the sex dwindles the touching, contact, and intimacy subsides.

Sexual happiness plays a big role in our level of commitment to another individual. Let us look at the role of commitment.

COMMITMENT – STEP SIX

The preoccupation with mate selection preoccupies a great deal of our adult lives. Social scientists call this the move from isolation to intimacy, where we select the appropriate partner in an attempt to create a safe haven from which to explore the world of adulthood. However, what is it that attracts a couple to move beyond passion, to intimacy and then to commitment?

Moving from casual dating to commitment (marriage or cohabitation) usually involves a number of stages. These include feelings of attachment and belonging, shared problem solving and disclosing of feelings. As the relationship moves closer toward intimacy there is a feeling of wanting to be committed. Without intimacy, true, deep-loving commitment never takes place.

However, it's important to note that individuals do commit to marriage without intimacy. These are the marriages or commitments that are based upon need and not desire. There are many reasons that we get into relationships, including loneliness, needing to settle down, stability, financial security, and regular sex.

Being committed from a place of unconditional love — which is sacred — is something we need to learn. Being committed for all the other reasons is based upon fear.

Fear is a strong motivator and is the basis behind most unsuccessful commitments. We commit to escape from our self-imposed emptiness. We settle for what appears to be love; all the time, in the back of our minds, knowing that we are entering into a union based upon unmet needs. Everyone who has entered into a commitment with the thoughts of need versus desires knows, deep inside, the reasons why they end up either failing in the relationship or are dreadfully unhappy.

Anyone who has been in a relationship that has failed has had one or more of the following thoughts:

- I'm tired and lonely.
- This may be the best I can do.
- She/he will make a good wife/husband.
- I need stability.
- I can always get a divorce.
- Somehow I'll get out of this.
- I want to have children and the clock is ticking.
- She/he comes from a good family.
- My family will accept this person.
- I need to escape and be taken care of.

None of these are reasons of love and erotic satisfaction. We believe that these are legitimate reasons for marrying an individual and, without knowledge of what it takes to keep each other satisfied and interested, we move into the most important decision of our lives. But we are set up to fail. For most of us, this sense of failure hits hard. It can cause us to question all of our decisions and choices in life.

However, even when we love with passion, intimacy, and commitment, there is no guarantee that consummate love will endure. Enduring relationships take work and commitment to the partnership, which means commitment to the satisfaction and happiness of each other. Sex, affection, intimacy, communication, compatibility, and erotic passion are all elements that must be part of a successful union. Honesty with yourself, as to your reasons for commitment should be the guiding factor. Again, the *Kama Sutra* states man/woman should consider compatibility before making love and making a commitment. The ancient sages taught that virtue (integrity and honesty), interest or attraction, and pleasure must be the basis for a successful and satisfying relationship.

Commitment in terms of life goals involves decision-making. The process involves having clearly defined goals and a plan for realizing those goals. This is the difference between reaching a goal and living in a dream. When you declare a goal with conviction, you are claiming that you have the self- confidence and commitment to make it happen. You decide to follow through, no matter what, until the dream becomes a reality. So it is with a relationship.

Unfortunately most people enter into life's process with unclear goals, conflict, negative conditioning, and a lack of commitment. This of course is the path to failure. This is why many people end up living their whole lives in situations that do not make them happy or give them fulfillment. They accept what comes their way, especially in a relationship, and stay for reasons other than love.

Relationships are no different from any other of life's goals. Because no one tells us that we can also choose the type of relationship we desire and meet it with passion and intensity, most people settle for what appears, on the surface, to be a good relationship. Without the passion and strength of conviction to make it successful, full commitment can never take place. Both parties must be committed to the necessary work that it takes to keep the relationship vibrant and alive. This begins with knowledge and understanding of what it means to find sacred love and what it means to experience that love through the passion of erotic pleasures.

To create the sacred, passionate, erotic vessel of a relationship, we learn to surrender our attachments and demands and learn to love by letting go of expectations and, instead, working to keep the relationship interesting.

This, of course, means we need to be open, trusting and committed. It is openness, trust and commitment that create the sacred vessel from which we find the freedom to grow and experience true love within a relationship.

Once we come together with another person with the intention of creating a sacred love relationship, the following guidelines will help us to stay focused on the deeper spiritual aspect of the relationship.

1. Always practice telling and hearing the truth. Truth means conducting our actions, words, and thoughts in accordance with the truth. We are truthful when thoughts, words, and actions are in harmony. If we are angry then our thoughts, words, and actions, will reflect this truth; just as if we are peaceful our thoughts, words, and actions will reflect calmness. Games and lies lead only to anger, fear, and mistrust. Being forthright whether it brings pleasure or pain will always lead to the highest good. The truth should always be revealed with one caveat: no intention to harm.

2. Stay in the present moment. Try always to stay with the experience of the moment rather than slipping into some intellectual fabrication of what we are feeling and experiencing. Whether pleasure or pain, stay in the moment and express the truth.

3. Accept the relationship as it is. Do not enter into a relationship with the aim of changing another person. If you cannot accept the nuances of another, there will surely be conflict. Everyone comes with some baggage. It is up to each of us to assess the baggage and give it acceptance or move out of the relationship. To stay will bring resentment, anger, and turmoil.

4. Respect and appreciate yourself, your partner, and the relationship. The ability to find true love begins with a sense of self- respect. Without a respect for self, we fall too easily in that insecure place where we become blind to the pitfalls of an unhealthy relationship. When we show respect and appreciation for our love and our relationships, we have the opportunity to experience the fullness and uniqueness of an intimate love affair. In the wholeness, we will find liberation beyond anything imaginable.

5. Recognize that a relationship has the ability to reflect back to you both positive and negative aspects of yourself. Recognizing this, we become a little more solid and accepting and cease to blame others for what is simply a reflection of us.

6. Share your passion and your fears. Be open in your communication with each other, sharing both your greatest desires and passions and your greatest fears and apprehensions. This creates open communication, which is paramount to a healthy balanced relationship.

7. Stop trying to impose an agenda onto the relationship. Oftentimes, we enter into a relationship and immediately begin to want structure and knowing. We lose the ease and Zen-like ability to let the relationship unfold on its own. In the Zen moment of love we have the opportunity to experience the purity of love without any self-imposed agenda.

8. Practice forgiveness. Be willing to forgive another for something that may have hurt you. Oftentimes, the hurt was unintentional. Sometimes it is best to simply let go.

9. Be playful, laugh, and have fun. Take time to enjoy the relationship and simply have fun and laughter in the moment. Play is one of the key elements to love and sexual satisfaction.

10. Schedule time to be alone and quiet with each other. Quiet times without any agenda allow a couple to explore inner passions and peaceful thoughts.

11. Honor the need to share interest, friends, and work, as well as the need for each person to have separateness. We all need times of separation and times of union.

12. Explore within the relationship the connection of spirituality to sexuality. Look carefully at your attitude towards sexuality. Do you use sex to grow and become whole or do you use it to control another person out of your own insecurity and fear? Sexuality has the potential to open us up to the deeper spiritual aspect of ourselves where the sexual experience is far beyond the world of everyday sex.

Using these guidelines, we can begin to make our relationships sacred and loving. Through intimacy, we learn to be supportive, compassionate, and authentic. We all want to be loved, to give love, to be accepted, and to accept unconditionally. When we use openness, truth, and commitment to create the vessel of relationship, we create a safe haven for the healthy nurturing of a sacred love.

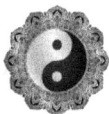

*~ A successful life: grow old gracefully with wisdom
and a sense of humor. ~*

THE SEVEN - DAY PLAN

So now that we have looked at the theoretical aspects of sexuality and relationships, let us look at a practical plan for implementing what we've learned. Let us create some sexual energy. The best sexual energy is a balance of desire and passion. It begins within you. Whether you are looking to bring love into your life or want to improve the love in your life, creative sexuality with a hint of magic will bring you all you desire. First, you must be absolutely sure of what you want and be willing to stay focused, no matter how long it takes. The more focused and determined you are, the quicker things will happen.

I'm going to give you a seven-day plan to get you started. However, you must believe with absolute faith that you will receive the object of your desire. So first, you must fixate on exactly what you want to draw into your life. The seven-day plan is to get you started. It will present you with tools that you can use and must use beyond the seven days to draw love and erotic sacred sex into your life — and for that matter, anything else you might desire. There are no shortcuts but if followed, this plan will work. However, remember when following this plan, that your own plan may need to be adjusted, and depending upon where you are in your life, there may be obstacles you need to overcome. Do not look for immediate results. The secret to manifesting our desires is to learn first to direct our own energy and, second, master ourselves. We must remember that we are body, mind and soul plugged into the entire universe. What happens on one side of the world affects all of us. We are not isolated. We all have the power to make things happen. It begins with a belief in the power to create.

The physicist Fritjof Capra refers to the universe as a complicated web of relations that unify into a whole. He explains that everything affects everything. Therefore, whatever you project from your mind has the power to affect many things at many levels. Your thoughts have a definite impact on the external world. However, this ability to project and influence is something that must be learned. We must first learn to slip through the barriers of the mind that prevent us from both sending and receiving information. There is a solution to every problem. We can move from a lower plane of thinking to a higher plane. We can lift our troubles and difficulties to precise vantage points where we become an active, rather than passive, facilitator with the power to change any situation. But remember, no event ever creates another event out of nothing. Each event is a crossroad that interchanges with all the other events in the universe. Our consciousness is not limited by space and time. Therefore, we can create and project and, in due time, expect to receive.

Remember our brain waves? Beta, alpha, theta, and delta. The brain waves, you will recall, are different states of consciousness — beta being fully awake and delta being our sleep state. We create in the alpha state, which is a state of deep meditation. First, fix in your mind exactly what you desire. You must be very clear and have total belief. Start with a notebook or your portable computer, something you carry with you throughout the day. You will need to keep notes. Write the date and then write out your desire. For example, I want to bring back the love and erotic sex between my lover and myself, or I want to find my true lover. Define what you want to happen between you and your lover or what you want your lover to be like. Be realistic, be precise, and have complete faith. Next, we need to move into alpha state.

Alpha state and the third eye are associated with the sixth chakra in yoga. It is the area between the eyebrows in the center of the forehead. When the third eye is in balance, we master our minds and pierce the veil of illusion. Our awareness is focus, with a meditative mind and an ability to know the unknown and see the unseen. Science tells us that this third eye spot is associated with the pineal gland. The pineal gland is how we receive light. Anatomists believe that the gland is a remnant of the third eye that never developed through evolution. Throughout history, culture after culture has made reference to the all-knowing third eye.

We need to spend a little time on this first part of the plan because it is essential to manifesting your desires. The pineal gland is located in the center of the brain. It is affected by light. It's associated with the sixth chakra in yoga where prophecy and increased psychic awareness of consciousness ascends.

This pineal gland controls the various biorhythms of the body. It works in harmony with the hypothalamus gland, which directs the body's thirst, hunger, sexual desire, and the biological clock that determines our aging process.

While the physiological function of the pineal gland has been unknown until recent times, mystical traditions and esoteric schools have long known this area in the middle of the brain to be the connecting link between the physical and spiritual worlds. Considered the most powerful and highest source of ethereal energy available to humans, the pineal gland has always been important in initiating supernatural powers. Development of psychic talents has been closely associated with this organ of higher vision.

By closing our eyes and breaking the component colors of light into the seven primary colors, we can lower our brain waves from beta to alpha. It's much like when we are lost in daydreaming, doodling, listening to music, or meditating. Remember, the vibrational energy of light and color have many therapeutic effects on the body-mind.

The easiest way to reach alpha is through a meditation that is a yoga countdown of the colors of the chakras or energy centers that make up your being. Read this section several times before you attempt to do it, as you do not want to stop in the middle of the meditation to reread the instructions.

Find a quiet place and then lie down on your yoga mat, a towel, or a blanket. Close your eyes and take in three deep, long breaths. Relax. Now focus your energy on your third eye located between your eyebrows. Clear your mind, and visualize a clear empty space filled only with the color of indigo (blue-black). Keep in mind that you do not need to have your eyes open to see. You can also see through the mind's eye.

Now, in your mind's eye see the color red. Take in a deep breath and release.

Now, the color orange. Take in a deep breath and release.

Now, the color yellow. Take in a deep breath and release.

Now, the color green. Take in a deep breath and release.

Now, the color blue. Take in a deep breath and release.

And now, indigo again. Take in three deep breaths and release.

Notice that these are the colors of the chakras or energy centers that go up and down the spine. In yoga, we work to open and balance these important centers, tapping into our intuitive selves.

Now, pull up to a sitting position (keeping your eyes closed) and sit back on your heels with your hands interlaced and resting on your chest. Clear your mind and take in three deep breaths. Drop your hands into your lap with the palms up and say to yourself, I am bringing health and love into my life. This will clear away any negative energy. Open your eyes slowly, and allow the moment to unfold.

This meditation can be done every day, but since we are focusing on a seven-day plan, do this meditation every day for the next seven days. Take a few minutes in the morning before you start your day. First, think about what it is you want to accomplish most, and then quietly slip into the meditation.

Self-esteem and proper self-love are necessary for successful, happy, and healthy living. A prerequisite for all success is a belief that you deserve to have personal wealth, health, and love in your life. With wealth, health, and love in your life, you have so much more to share with others. Therefore, every "I believe" must be turned into an "I know." It is one thing to believe and quite another to know with complete certainty that you will receive that which you desire.

Most important, all instinctive and intuitive power should be used to elicit your desires in a gentle and loving manner. You cannot control and overpower another person. You should never try to force a situation or create unhappiness. If you do unhappiness will come back to you three times over.

This meditation and the steps in the book will not automatically bring you that which you desire. Remember, the time must be right, and the right amount of energy must be created. Everything has its time. The question is, when the time is right, will you be there? Therefore, it is important that you keep your focus no matter what. When the time is right, if you are prepared, it will all come together.

Now let's recap so far:

Each day you will read to yourself your written desire.

Then you will take a few moments and go into alpha meditation.

And then capture a moment of quietude by sitting up, closing your eyes, and taking in three deep breaths.

Next, each morning, you will do the magic mirror exercise. Self-love means being able to truly look at yourself and love what you see reflecting back. Your mirror is your reflection, and, like all reflections, if you truly focus, you will be able to see the beauty beneath the surface. Folklore, legend, and fairy tales are full of stories about magic mirrors. Your bathroom mirror is a great place to gaze at yourself each morning to give self-love. When you brush your teeth, put on makeup, comb your hair, wash your face, or shave, look deep into the reflection past the image, and say, "I love you, you are terrific, you are beautiful, you can accomplish anything you desire, because you're special."

This exercise may sound silly, but it is essential. Say it with full conviction, intention, and purpose. If you are self-conscious about other people hearing you, close the door. There is nothing wrong with taking a little time to love yourself. Pay attention to your self-consciousness and let it be a guide. It may reflect back to you what is hindering you from radiating out the kind of energy that attracts people to you. Practice this mirror exercise every day. Continue even after you have found the love of your life. It will reinforce your relationships and bring appreciation and love into your life.

You love yourself; now make yourself beautiful. Men and women have always adorned themselves to attract the opposite sex. Paint, tattoos, makeup, and jewelry date back to ancient times. The use of color affects our behavior, emotions, and dispositions. Animals employ color to attract mates and so do humans. How you present yourself to the world says a lot about you. Highly sexual beings are usually very well groomed, making use of color and adornment to attract lovers.

The tracing out of the eye to make one seem more radiant and mysterious is a time-honored custom. Goddesses, such as Ishtar, Maat, and Mari, were portrayed with finely outlined eyes to reflect their magic and ability to see all, know all, and illuminate the world. Your makeup or lack thereof says a lot about you. Keep it natural but do accentuate your most notable feature. Pay close attention to the eyes, for they are truly the gateway to the soul.

Jewelry is also a very important part of drawing love into your life. Make it tasteful and interesting. Use stones and crystals as well as gold and silver. Always wear something that attracts light and stands out, so it will draw attention to you.

The way you dress is crucial to attracting a lover. Each day for the next seven days, pay close attention to how you dress. You don't need to dress to the hilt. But remember, each day people evaluate how you are dressed and how you look. You never know whom you are going to meet or run into. The way you are dressed gives the first impression of the person inside the clothes. You always want the way you look to reflect the person inside you. If you are looking for love and want to enhance your sexuality, you need to "put it out there." Not in a sleazy, low-class manner, but discretely with class. You don't need a lot of money, but you do need to be creative. I learned a long time ago how to make a silk purse out of a sow's ear. If you have never heard this expression, it means to take something of seemingly worthless value and turn it into something beautiful. Remember alchemy, the ability to turn something seemingly useless into gold?

Throughout most of my life, money was a struggle. When I was a child, my grandmother would bring my mother material and patterns from which to make me dresses and coats. I had beautifully handmade dresses made from leftover material, buttons, and trim. I watched my mother turn relatively little into something creative. As I matured, I developed a love for design and clothes. I loved putting colors and textures together and creating, in my mind, a mix and match of things from my closet. I would retreat to my bedroom and spend hours creating my school week's outfits. I wanted to be a fashion designer, but was quickly told that it would be impossible. New York was a dangerous place, and I did not have the talent to compete. I never lost that dream. I just kept making outfits out of whatever I had at hand. I taught myself to use accessories and scarves. I bought classic clothes of the best quality I could afford and wildly dressed them up with jewelry, scarves, shoes, and belts. In other words, I developed a wardrobe of my own style. I learned to make a silk purse out of a sow's ear.

Dress carefully and pay attention to your mood. Adorn yourself and embrace all those little imperfections. Stop focusing on what you can't wear and can't do and focus on what you can. Always dress neatly and cleanly because, as my parents used to say, "Cleanliness is next to godliness, and just because someone is poor, they don't need to be dirty." I took those things to heart and I believe them to be true. A clean person is a lot sexier than someone who does not care about his or her appearance. Even if your body is not perfect by Hollywood standards, you can still dress with flare and have fun.

As you become more self-confident and connected to your own identity, you should dress to send out signals about who you are. If you feel drawn to a certain era, certain colors, and certain styles, wear them. Use colors to highlight your best features and to downplay unflattering ones.

Each day, get up and pay attention to your mood. Are you playful, serious, sporty, bohemian, intellectual...who are you today, and how can you best personify yourself with a hint of sexual allure? Add a talisman such as a feather, a headband, earrings, beads, or a ring. Make it something that is a statement about you.

For example, as I write this, I am wearing amber jewelry that I bought in Prague. Wearing amber, according to folklore, is believed to bring love, luck, strength, healing, and protection into your life. Amber calms stressed nerves and hyperactivity. Wearing amber, you may find humor and joy. Legend has it that amber provided sorcerers and magicians with enhanced powers.

Earrings were first used as talismans to keep evil spirits out of one's head. To me, earrings are one of the cheapest and best ways to enhance an outfit. If you shop carefully, you can always find fun earrings to set off your mood. Each day wear some special piece of jewelry. Allow yourself to be drawn to the right piece.

Adorning yourself means to connect with your inner essence. Know who you are and what you want to project, and then put yourself together in the very best way to express it. Don't try to copy another person's style. It will not work. You need to find your own special look. This will draw to you a lover who matches you and appreciates your style.

Here is something very important in the game of love, sex, and attraction. If you do not like the style of the person you are with, it will become a problem. As much as you must project your own sense of style, you must pay attention to a potential mate's style. It says so much about how you view the world. Compatibility is very high up on the successful relationship scale, and compatible styles are very important. You must be attracted to the way a person looks and dresses. That does not mean that the person needs to be classically beautiful or handsome. It simply means you know if you are attracted to what you see. If so, you have style and look compatible.

Remember, you cannot change the style and look of another person. You can enhance it but never totally change a person's sense of style, because that is how they related to and look at the world. On one level, it is unique to each of us. It says a lot about how we envision the world.

Don't forget about adding color to your look. The colors of love are the shades of pink and orange. Green will bring balance. Blues makes you more cerebral and purples enlighten your spirit. Each one of the colors will draw an energy to you either because you are wearing one of them or you are drawn to one of them. Pay attention to the colors that you are drawn to throughout the week. Pinks and oranges align with the sacral chakra, which is the center of sexuality. When they draw you in, you may feel a warmth and a sensual "hello." Green may bring a sense of balance to your life, and that may be just what you need to bring love into your life. Blue will affect your thinking process and perhaps open your mind, which may be closed and prejudice, keeping you from finding a lover. Or maybe the shades of purple will draw you in, lifting your spirits and making you a little more playful and appreciative and willing to live life with passion. Keep these colors in mind throughout the week.

So, each day for the next seven days, read your desire, do the alpha meditation, do the magic mirror speech, make yourself up to be natural, accentuating your best features with a bit of flair, wear carefully chosen clothes, pay attention to color, and add adornment. Be very aware of each choice you make. In other words, for the next seven days, focus on the task. Consciously think about how you dress and how you look.

Our scent says so much about us. In a subconscious way, our natural individual scents draw a person to us. On a very subtle level, the natural pheromones spark attraction. Because the human pheromones are so indistinguishable, being clean and natural is a wonderful palette from which to add a scent. Nothing smells worse than body odor, cigarette smoke, and dirt mixed with perfume. It's also terrible when scents such as soap or deodorant clash with each other.

The way to a lover's heart is most assuredly through the nose. The ability of scents to affect our moods has been well-documented using aromatherapy. Each day, wear a perfume that contains one or more of the following scents: jasmine, vanilla, sandalwood, ylang-ylang, clary sage, or rose. Do not overpower the fineness of the scent by adding too much. You might burn a candle of beeswax (the best conduit for true essential oils) that contains one of these scents. Spray the bed and sheets with an aromatherapy spray. Always use a good-quality essential oil. Oils are often cut and artificial, so make sure you buy from a reputable essential oil company. If the oil from the bottle stains a piece of cloth, it probably has been cut, which means it is not pure. Good-quality perfumers like Thierry Mugler, Hermes, Chanel, Boucheron, and Cartier use top-quality oils in their perfumes.

Here is a natural lover's potion to scent your house: simmer in a cup or two of natural spring water, a tablespoon of salt, apple peelings, a sprig of clove, and a cinnamon stick with just a drop or two of patchouli oil or musk. Let the aroma fill the house. Put a few drops on your lover's pillow, a doorknob or on a chair. Leave the scent discreetly in carefully chosen places.

Music always sets the mood. If your intention is to enhance your sexuality, then music that sets the mood is necessary. Listen to the following music throughout the week. All of these songs can be downloaded and made into a playlist at iTunes. You can also make your own list. Go through your old CDs, tapes, or records and take out music that makes you feel sexy. Dedicate at least 15 minutes a day listening to this music.

Music to set the mood:

1. I Want to Hold Your Hand/Beatles
2. Be My Lover/Various Artists
3. Do Ya Think I'm Sexy/Remix Rod Stewart
4. Burning Love/Elvis Presley
5. I've Been Thinking About You/Londonbeat
6. Hanky Panky/Dynamix
7. Let's Get It On/Marvin Gaye
8. Cosmic Love/Florence + the Machine
9. My Girl/The Temptations
10. More Than Ever/Zoot Woman
11. Let's Stay Together/Al Green
12. At Last/Etta James

Create your own list of loving and sexy music. Check out my online yoga/dance class where, once a week, I will create a new music playlist. The class will work your sexy body-mind. Or check out my monthly playlist on my website http://www.doctorlynn.com. Remember, the same chemical burst of endorphins that makes up our orgasms is the same that we feel when we get up and dance. Aerobic exercise/dance is a great way to stay in shape and improve your sex life.

Music makes us feel sexy, romantic, and sensual. Dance is an art form and a form of lovemaking. It is the nonverbal expression of your moods and emotions. Movements and gestures communicate sexual rhythm. As you allow the music and the dance to overtake you and unravel your inner being, you will become the dance. Let yourself go. The dance of lovers has always provoked sexuality. Start by letting different parts of your body move with the music until you have released all tension. Relax and enjoy. Dance, exercise, and a healthy diet make for healthier people; and healthier people have better sex!

The British Medical Journal notes that a healthy lifestyle, which includes exercise, enhances performance in the bedroom. Healthier people have more and better sex!

Recap: Each day, repeat your desire to yourself. Go into alpha meditation, do the magic mirror, use sensual scents in your house and on your person, make yourself up, wear interesting outfits carefully chosen that portray the right message, adorn yourself with interesting jewelry, surround yourself with color and music, do Doctor Lynn's Xercise for a Sexy Body-Mind daily, and dance and listen to music or join me online for 60 minutes of sexy fun.

Now, one more magical task. This one I can tell you absolutely works, but it takes patience and faith. Get a clear rose crystal. Bathe it in sea salt and spring water and then wrap it in a white cloth and leave it for 24 hours. This will cleanse it and neutralize all unwanted vibrations and energies. Unwrap the crystal, and place it in the palm of your hand. Wrap your fingers around it. Close your eyes, and ask that the lover who is correct and good for you come into your life. This can be directed toward someone you love or someone you hope comes into your life. However, always ask for the crystal power to bring to you a good person who is correct for you. Wrap the crystal in pink, copper, red, or green cloth and tie it into a bundle with the same color ribbon or string. Carry it with you in your purse or pocket. I used pink cloth and, at the right time, a lover who was correct and good for me stepped into my life.

Now before you think I have stepped too far off the edge, *Scientific American* reported that scientists are trying to harness photonic crystals to use to function as circuits in communication and computing devices. You probably use items every day that contain LCD or liquid crystal displays — your plasma TV, computer, iPod, iPhone, watches, microwave ovens, and on, *ad infinitum.*

A crystal is a solid mass, containing silica. The majority of optic fibers made for telecommunication are made from silica. In other words, science is getting closer and closer to harnessing the conductivity of crystals.

Exactly three years before I met my now husband I did this exact crystal ritual. Now you may say, three years is a long time to wait. However, at the time, I was not ready and neither was my husband. I wanted to bring into my life a person who was correct and good for me. Over the three years, I worked on my writing, teaching, and my personal self. It was a very good time of tremendous growth. I carried the crystal with me in my purse for three years. When the time was right, my husband and I met; and he was the correct person, bringing love and prosperity into my life.

I believe in the power of communication, both as we understand it and as the power to use the energy of the mind to project and attract. Even Einstein believed that, beyond what we could comprehend as humans, there was an unknown energy or force. The laws of thermodynamics state that energy is never lost, it simply changes form.

A crystal meditation is one way to use the power of the mind through the medium of a natural transmitter to bring about desired results.

Now that we have looked at how to apply the natural sciences, it is time to put together a seven-day eating plan that emphasizes a diet for love, lust, sex, and more.

For the next seven days, follow these prescribed steps. You will be building up your energy and culminating this process by a sexual and sensual love feast on the seventh day. Even if you have not yet found your lover, make the feast for yourself. It is good practice and gets you ready for the time when he or she enters into your life. I hope that you will make several of these dietary steps part of your everyday routine. These will get you on the pathway to a healthy lifestyle, because a healthy happy soul is a sexy being and a sexy being will bring sensual pleasure into your life. Remember, part of finding love is being ready for it when it arrives. Otherwise, it can walk right past you.

Start your morning with a cup of green or white tea. There is a debate about which is better for your health. Green tea gives you a bit more of a caffeine kick while white tea delivers slightly more antioxidants. Either way, healthy tea is a great way to start your day. If you don't drink tea or coffee in the morning, try a cup of warm water with a little lemon or add a dropper full of Damiana's Nectar. You can also add Damiana's Nectar to your hot green or white tea. If you don't want the alcohol (which is minimal) from the nectar, put a dropper full in hot water or hot tea and the alcohol will evaporate, leaving a pure herbal essence.

Try giving up coffee for one week. Although coffee does have antioxidants, it is harsher than tea. If you need to sweeten the tea, add a little honey.

Breakfast should be light. Remember, this is not a diet but, rather, healthy foods to build and strengthen your sexual being. Start with Cleopatra's love drink. Supposedly, this drink made her a strong lover. It's healthy, strength- building, and full of aphrodisiac fruits.

Freeze peeled bananas cut in half. You will use half a banana each day. Place a few small ice cubes and the frozen banana in a blender. Add 1/2 cup of watermelon, 1/3 cup of papaya, 1/4 cup of orange juice, 1/4 cup of kefir or unflavored yogurt, a dash of ground cloves, and a dash of ground cinnamon. Blend to make a smooth drink.

If you need a little more substance to your breakfast, add a small bowl of oatmeal, sprinkled on top with a little cinnamon. Or have a piece of whole wheat bread with strawberry jam.

At midmorning, have a snack of dates and an apple. Remember, it was Eve who gave Adam the apple, opening his eyes to the pleasure of sexuality. The therapeutic value of both apples and dates has been well-documented. Apples are chock-full of nutrients and great for digestive disorders. Dates are strength-building and great for people who participate in strenuous physical activity. That means both are a great fuel to ignite the sexual fires.

For lunch and dinner, here is a list of erotic foods to mix and match. The idea is to become familiar with these foods so you can add them to your everyday meals. For example, when choosing rice, go for brown rice because it is high in vitamin B5. Vitamin B5 raises histamine levels, which is the neurotransmitter that increases arousal.

So eat liver, peanuts, lentils, brown rice, whole wheat, salmon, broccoli, grapes, tropical foods, citrus, cherries, cabbage, parsley, melons, and peppers. Do not forget niacin for that tingling feeling: sesame seeds, lean beef, barley, split peas, shrimp, haddock, eggs, peaches, tomatoes, and carrots.

Vitamin B6 for estrogen and testosterone: kidney beans, lima beans, chicken, fish, eggs, spinach, peas, avocado, tuna, hazelnuts, bananas, Brussels sprouts, sweet potatoes, and cauliflower.

Leafy greens, soybeans, and tofu enhance estrogen, the "come and get me" hormone. Vitamin E is an antioxidant that has been linked to improving sex drive. It is also found in salmon, legumes, brown rice, tofu, leafy greens, and soybeans.

Zinc and selenium are found in seafood, oysters, milk, oats, black beans, liver, anchovies, and eggs. Zinc and selenium are the minerals a man uses when he ejaculates, so give your man plenty of zinc-enhancing foods.

The sex brain also needs to be fed. It needs potassium, which can be found in bananas, sweet potatoes, tomatoes, and dairy products.

Don't forget to add dark chocolate to your diet. One piece of dark chocolate a day should be eaten. Don't overindulge, but do enjoy the sensual pleasure of chocolate. To get an extra kick of chocolate, take a dropper full of Damiana's Nectar each day. These sensually enhancing herbs in chocolate and honey will lift your mood and enhance your senses.

Add figs, asparagus, shiitake mushrooms, arugula, strawberries, onions, garlic, watercress, vanilla, marjoram, cinnamon, cloves, basil, black pepper, honey, wine, and beer to your grocery list. Choose from this variety of healthy sensual foods each day, carefully preparing fresh foods to delight your taste buds and ignite your sexual fires.

Purchase a bottle of Strega, an Italian potion of liqueur and herbs. Strega is long believed to be an aphrodisiac. *Strega* is the Italian word for "witch." It originates from the Benevento region of Italy, well known for witchcraft. Strega was said to be brewed originally as a witch's potion.

Strega can be purchased in any good wine store, or search online. Strega will be used in a recipe I will give you for a romantic honey cake.

In England, mead, which is made from honey, was considered an aphrodisiac. It was drunk for a month after the wedding to make a couple sexually potent. This is the origin of the word *honeymoon*. Damiana's Nectar is a combination of honey, chocolate, herbs, and alcohol taken in part from the ancient recipe for mead.

Read the list and get your provisions ahead of time. For the next seven days, you'll eat from the list, following certain guidelines and ending with a love feast on the seventh night.

The guidelines are:

1. Each day, make Cleopatra's love drink for breakfast.

2. Each day, have one dropper full of Damiana's nectar, either straight or diluted in a cup of tea or warm water. You can also dilute it into a bottle of cold water and sip throughout the day. (Optional).

3. Each day, eat one good-quality, dark, rich chocolate.

4. Each day, drink either Casanova's or Don Juan's cocktail in the afternoon.

5. Choose from the erotic food and herb-spice list for your foods to eat.

6. Remove all fast food, prepared foods, and canned or frozen foods. Eat fresh foods.

7. As you prepare each meal, do so with love and care.

8. Reread the chapter on spices and herbs. Make use of these in the foods you cook.

9. Remove junk food and soft drinks.

10. The last night, prepare the love feast.

Following these guidelines will introduce you to the world of sensual tastes and smells. At the same time, it will build up your sexual and sensual energy, which will emanate from your being and be cast out into the world. Share this with a loved one, or do it on your own and experience the sexual delight of nature's aphrodisiacs.

SAMPLE MENU

Here is a sample of a day's menu to get you started, along with a few recipes. Be creative. Just think about what you're eating and what you are using to spice your food.

Breakfast:
Start with green tea or hot water. Next, make Cleopatra's love drink.

In a blender, place ; half a frozen banana, a few ice cubes, 1/2 cup watermelon, 1/4 cup papaya, 1/4 cup of orange juice, dash of ground cloves, a dash of ground cinnamon, and 1/4 cup non-flavored yogurt or non-flavored kefir. Blend and drink.

Midmorning: two dates, an apple and a dropper of Damiana's Nectar straight from the bottle or diluted in hot water and cold water.

Lunch: Dark, leafy, mixed greens, sliced tomatoes, and egg salad on whole wheat bread or a bowl of split-pea soup with whole grain roll, a salad of dark leafy greens, tomatoes, mushrooms, and cottage cheese with a little honey mustard dressing. For a vegetarian lunch, have tofu, greens, and vegetables as a salad or stir-fry. Grapes and figs for dessert. Tea or water to drink.

Mid-afternoon: If you haven't had your dropper full of Damiana's Nectar, this would be a great time. Remember either straight or diluted. One chunk of dark, rich chocolate.

Late afternoon cocktail: Casanova and Don Juan were known for their lovemaking. Supposedly, they drank these two cocktails on a regular basis. Drink either one or switch one for one day and one for the next.

Don Juan: In an eight-ounce glass, pour tomato juice and add a tablespoon of crushed fresh basil. Stir vigorously and drink.

Casanova: Fill 3/4 of an eight-ounce glass with steamed apple juice. Fill to the top with fresh grapefruit juice. Add a dash of cinnamon and a dash of cloves. Mix and drink.

Dinner should be fish, chicken, or meat. Again, if a vegetarian, use erotic vegetables and tofu, beans, or lentils with brown rice, and make a stir-fry.

Poached or broiled salmon with a spinach avocado salad is a good choice. Or broil a steak or chicken. Serve sweet potatoes, Brussels sprouts, and asparagus. Carrots and cauliflower are also good choices. Make dill sauce with non-flavored yogurt and fresh chopped dill weed. Add a crusty bread and olive oil for dipping.

NATURALLY SEXY & HEALTHY ~ Doctor Lynn Wylnn

Serve a good quality wine or a sparkling nonalcoholic cider. Finish the meal with a simple dessert — like fruit, sorbet, or a little chocolate.

In the evening, if you need a little snack, make it something light made with milk or yogurt so that you get a good night's sleep. Make healthy choices from the list of ingredients given. The seventh night will be a love feast.

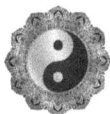

RECIPES

The following are some recipes to try, and then we will put together the final night's love feast.

BREAKFAST

ASPARAGUS AND TOMATO OMELET

Makes 2 servings

3 eggs, beaten
1/4 cup of nonfat cottage cheese
1/3 cup of raw blanched asparagus tips
1 medium tomato, sliced

In a blender or food processor, at medium to high speed, whip eggs and cottage cheese.

Heat a skillet with a drizzle of olive oil and pour in the egg mixture. Stir until set.

Turn onto a serving plate and arrange asparagus tips and sliced tomatoes on top of the eggs.

THREE - GRAIN PEANUT BUTTER BREAD

Makes 8 servings
Tastes great sliced, toasted, and served with honey.

Preheat oven to 350 degrees
1/2 cup of cornmeal
1/2 cup of oatmeal
1 cup of whole wheat or any other whole grain flour
3 teaspoons of baking powder
1/2 teaspoon of cinnamon
1/3 cup of peanut butter
2 egg whites
1 teaspoon of safflower oil or olive oil
1 tablespoon of nonfat yogurt
2 packets of stevia
1 cup of cold water

In a bowl, combine cornmeal, oatmeal, flour, baking powder, and cinnamon. Add stevia, peanut butter, egg whites, yogurt, and oil. Mix with a fork until blended.

Add water and mix thoroughly. Place in nonstick loaf pan and cook for 30 minutes.

Allow to cool, removing from pan and serve or cool and toast.

APPETIZERS

HUMMUS SPREAD

Makes 4 servings

This Middle Eastern spread is high in vegetable protein. Beans such as chickpeas are low in fat and high in potassium, iron, thiamine, and sodium. Beans are also a great source of complex carbohydrates. The digestive process of beans appears to release protease inhibitors, which scientists believe are extremely effective in blocking the formation of certain cancer cells including colon and breast cancer. L-arginine, an amino acid in garbanzos, provides nitric oxide, which widens blood vessels, helping to speed natural lubrication. Four tablespoons of hummus have the daily amount you need.

6 oz can of rinsed & drained chickpeas (garbanzo beans)
2 tablespoons of lemon juice
1 tablespoon of tahini (sesame paste)
1 teaspoon of olive oil
1 teaspoon of minced garlic
2 tablespoons of finely minced scallions
(green Dash of paprika and white portions)

In a food processor, combine all ingredients except scallions and paprika and process until pureed. Stir in scallions. Place in serving bowl and chill for 1 hour.

Sprinkle top with paprika. Serve with a salad atop greens and chopped vegetables or serve with slices of pita bread.

PESTO

Pesto is a great garnish for fish, chicken, or pasta. It also works well as a dip for raw vegetables.

1 cup of low-fat cottage cheese
1 cup of fresh basil leaves
2 tablespoons of grated Parmesan cheese
1 tablespoon of pine nuts or walnuts
2 garlic cloves, peeled (or the equivalent minced garlic)

In a food processor, combine all ingredients and process until smooth. Serve at room temperature or chill.

SALADS

WALDORF SALAD

Makes 4 servings

In many ancient cultures, the walnut was thought to bring good luck and good health. The Romans called the walnut the royal nut. The oil found in walnuts is one of the good fats, polyunsaturated fat that tends to lower cholesterol.

1 cup of plain organic nonfat yogurt

1/4 cup of reduced-fat nondairy mayonnaise

2 teaspoons of lemon juice

1 packet of stevia

4 small sweet apples, diced and peeled

1 cup of chopped celery

1 tablespoon of sunflower seeds

1/2 cup of chopped walnuts

SHREDDED BIBB LETTUCE

Place yogurt, mayonnaise, lemon juice, and stevia in a bowl and mix. Add remaining ingredients (except Bibb lettuce) and toss. Chill to blend flavors. Serve over Bibb lettuce.

MACHE SALAD (LAMB'S LETTUCE)

Makes 4 servings
4 ounces of mache lettuce
2 avocados, skinned, pitted, and cut into chunks
2 grapefruits peeled and sectioned. Drain and
reserve the juice
1/2 cup of roasted, chopped macadamia nuts (or use
almonds or walnuts)

CITRUS VINAIGRETTE

Whisk
1 tablespoon of grapefruit juice
1 tablespoon of lime juice
Grated zest of one lime
2 tablespoons of extra virgin olive oil
Dash of sea salt and a dash of black pepper vinaigrette
ingredients together. Toss with mache, avocado,
grapefruit sections, and toasted macadamia nuts.

LUNCH

BASIC TOFU SALAD

Makes three cups of salad.
1 pound of hard tofu
1 tablespoon of olive oil
1 teaspoon of fresh lemon juice
1 teaspoon of grated garlic
1/2 teaspoon of onion powder
1/4 cup of finely chopped parsley
1 teaspoon of mustard
Dash of sea salt and dash of black pepper

Chop the tofu finely and combine with the remaining ingredients. Let sit for 30 minutes and taste. Serve on a sandwich or on a bed of greens.

Optional additions:
1/4 cup chopped of dill pickle
1/4 cup of diced celery
1/4 cup of diced tomato
1 tablespoon of minced green onion
2 teaspoons of chopped capers
1 tablespoon of chopped olives
1/4 cup of chopped cilantro

MANGO LIME SALSA CHICKEN SALAD

Rub boneless chicken thigh or breast (8 ounces) with 1/2 teaspoon of chili powder and broil. Slice.

Combine 1 cup of diced fresh mango and 2 teaspoons each of honey, lime juice, and minced scallions.

Place sliced chicken over a bed of organic mixed greens and pour salsa over the top.

SOUPS

PUMPKIN CURRY SOUP

Makes 2 servings
1 small onion, finely chopped
1 small green pepper, finely chopped
1/2 of a 16-ounce can of unseasoned pumpkin puree
1 14.5-ounce can of chicken broth (or vegetable broth)
1 teaspoon of curry powder
2 tablespoons of fresh chopped parsley
1 teaspoon of olive oil
Nonfat plain yogurt
Crushed red pepper
In a medium saucepan over medium heat, sauté onion and pepper in olive oil for about 2 minutes. Add pumpkin

puree and chicken broth. Stir with wire whisk until smooth. Heat to boiling, stirring constantly. Stir in the curry and parsley. Pour into individual bowls. Place a tablespoon of yogurt in the center of each and swirl. Sprinkle the top with crushed red pepper.

COLD STRAWBERRY SOUP

Makes 4 Servings
1 quart of fresh or frozen strawberries
1/3 cup of orange juice
1/4 cup of cranberry juice
1/2 cup of yogurt
1 teaspoon of lime juice
2 tablespoons of sugar
1 tablespoon of cinnamon
1/4 teaspoon of nutmeg
Whipped cream or yogurt for garnish
Fruit for garnish
Fresh mint leaves for garnish
Mix all ingredients (except garnishes) together and puree in food processor or blender. Chill for several hours to allow flavors to blend.

Garnish each serving with a dollop of whipped cream or yogurt, more cinnamon if desired, fruit, and a mint leaf.

VEGETABLE DISHES

RATATOUILLE

Makes 4 servings

Ratatouille is a soup, as well as a vegetable dish. You can also add diced cooked chicken to make it a meat meal. Each of the vegetables in ratatouille have healing properties: zucchini is good for elimination and healthy skin; red pepper contains copious amounts of vitamin C, the anti-stress vitamin; and eggplant is considered to be the most powerful food for a woman as it is both energizing and soothing.

4 large scallions, diced (about 1/2 cup)
2 cloves of garlic, minced
1 medium eggplant, peeled
1 cup of fresh sliced mushrooms
1/2 cup of celery, chopped
2 large tomatoes, chopped
2 small zucchinis, sliced
1 sweet red pepper, diced
2 tablespoons of olive oil
1 teaspoon of basil
1 teaspoon of oregano
1 tablespoon of dry white wine
Dash of dried red pepper
Fresh grated Parmesan cheese

Sauté scallion and garlic in olive oil over medium heat. Stir in eggplant, mushrooms, and celery and cook for five minutes, stirring occasionally. Stir in tomatoes, zucchinis, scallions, oregano, basil, wine, and red pepper. Reduce heat to low and simmer for 15 minutes until eggplant is tender. Add a dash of dried red pepper.

Option:
Add 1 cup of diced cooked chicken or add 1 cup of canned red kidney beans. Serve over basmati rice. Serve in bowls topped with a little grated Parmesan cheese.

BAKED LENTILS WITH TOMATOES

Makes 4 servings
2 tablespoons of olive oil
1/2 cup of chopped onions
1/2 cup of chopped celery
1/2 cup of chopped green pepper
1 16-ounce can of tomatoes, chopped and drained
1/2 teaspoon of dried oregano
Dash of garlic powder
16 ounces of cooked lentils
2 tablespoons of wheat germ or dried breadcrumbs
1 tablespoon grated Parmesan cheese

Heat oil in pan. Add onion, celery, and green pepper and cook until tender. Preheat oven to 350 degrees.

Spray a 11/2-quart baking dish with a nonstick cooking spray. Combine onion mixture with tomatoes, oregano, garlic powder, and lentils. Mix well. Sprinkle top with wheat germ and Parmesan cheese. Bake uncovered for 30 minutes.

CAULIFLOWER TOFU BAKE

Makes 2 servings
Serve with a side salad of mixed greens and sliced tomatoes for a complete vegetarian meal. Note: You can use broccoli or any other vegetable.

1 medium head of fresh cauliflower — steam flowerets
6 ounces of soft tofu, drained and mashed
2 ounces of grated Parmesan cheese
1/4 cup of reduced-calorie Italian dressing
Nonstick cooking spray

Place cooked cauliflower in a 1-quart baking dish that has been sprayed with a nonstick cooking spray. Preheat oven to 375 degrees. In a small bowl, combine tofu, Parmesan cheese, and dressing. Mix well. Spoon over cauliflower. Bake for 20 minutes.

VEGGIE BURGER WITH PAPAYA SALSA

Makes 4 servings
1 16-ounce can of chickpeas (garbanzo beans),
1/4cup of minced cilantro
1 clove of garlic, minced
2 egg whites
1 teaspoon of sea salt
1/4 teaspoon of cayenne pepper
1/3 cup of whole wheat flour
2 tablespoons of olive oil drained

Process all ingredients, except for the flour, in a food processor or blender until combined. Place the flour on waxed paper. Drop a fourth of the mixture onto the flour, and using wet fingertips, gently shape into a patty.

Flip to coat the other side. Make three more patties. Heat the oil in a large nonstick skillet over medium heat and cook patties until golden on both sides.

Serve on whole-grain rolls with salsa.

SALSA

Makes 2 cups
2 plum tomatoes, sliced
1 papaya peeled, seeded, and diced
2 tablespoons of apple cider vinegar
1 tablespoon of honey
1 jalapeno pepper, seeded, minced 1 tablespoon of lemon juice.

Combine all ingredients.

CHICKEN DISHES

CHICKEN TOMASI

Makes 6 servings
This is an adaptation from a traditional Hungarian recipe, supposedly named after the town of Tomasi.

3 pounds of boneless, skinless chicken parts cut into bite-sized pieces
2 teaspoons of olive oil
1 medium onion, chopped
1 clove of garlic, finely chopped
3–5 teaspoons of paprika

1/4 teaspoon of cayenne pepper
1/2 cup of chicken broth
8-ounce container of nonfat plain yogurt
1/4 cup of low fat milk
Salt and pepper to taste.

Brown chicken in olive oil. Remove to a platter and drain on a paper towel. Sauté onion and garlic in the olive oil until tender. Return chicken to pan. Sprinkle with cayenne pepper and paprika. Pour in the broth. Simmer covered until chicken is tender, or about 20 minutes.

Remove pan from heat. Remove chicken with slotted spoon to a platter. Keep warm. Let sauce cool to lukewarm. Stir together in a bowl the yogurt and milk until smooth. Stir in a little of the lukewarm sauce. Stir yogurt mixture back into saucepan.

Place over low heat and add salt and pepper to taste. Return chicken to saucepan and gently reheat but do not boil.

Serve over rice or couscous, or with a dinner salad and fresh bread.

CURRY CHICKEN

Makes 4 servings
2/3 cup of nonfat, plain yogurt
2 cloves of minced garlic
1 1/2 teaspoons of curry powder
1/4 teaspoon of ground ginger
Dash of cayenne pepper
2 pounds of boneless, skinless chicken parts cut into chunks
1/2 cup of chopped fresh onion
1 1/2 cups of chopped fresh tomatoes
1 bay leaf
4 tablespoons of fresh chopped cilantro leaves
1 tablespoon of olive oil

Combine yogurt and spices in medium bowl. Add chicken parts and turn to coat. Let stand at room temperature for 30 minutes. Sauté onion in a skillet with olive oil until lightly brown. Add tomatoes and bay leaf. Lower heat and simmer for 5 minutes. Add chicken and yogurt mixture and stir to combine. Bring mixture back to a boil. Lower heat; cover and simmer, turning once or twice until chicken is tender, about 30 minutes.

Remove bay leaf and serve each serving with a topping of fresh chopped cilantro. Serve plain or over rice and vegetables.

APRICOT OR MARMALADE CHICKEN

Serves 6
12 chicken thighs
1 cup of apricot preserves or marmalade
1 cup of French dressing
1-ounce package of dry onion soup mix

Preheat oven to 350 degrees. In a medium bowl, combine the jam, dressing, and soup mix. Mix ingredients together. Place chicken pieces in a 9 x 13-inch baking dish. Pour apricot mixture over chicken and bake uncovered in the preheated oven for 50 to 60 minutes.

FISH

The fish recipes chosen here all supply a great source of Omega-3, the essential fatty acid. Use salmon or any solid fish. Halibut would be a good choice.

CHILLED POACHED SALMON

Makes 4 servings

3 cups of water
1 cup of white wine

1 lemon, sliced
1/4 cup of sliced scallions
1/4 teaspoon of sea salt and
1/4 teaspoon of black pepper
4 1-inch thick salmon steaks

In a large skillet, combine water, wine, lemon slices, scallions, salt, and pepper. Heat to boiling, add salmon steaks, and cover. Reduce heat to low. Simmer gently for 7 to 10 minutes. Remove fish from liquid. Cover and refrigerate until chilled.

SPICY SALMON DINNER

Makes 4 servings
Poach 4 salmon fillets as above recipe. While salmon is poaching, heat
1 tablespoon of olive oil and add
2 teaspoons of curry powder and sauté 15 seconds.

Add sliced scallions (2 bunches — bottoms only);
2 ripe pears, cored and sliced; and
1 red pepper, cut into julienne strips.

Place warm salmon on serving plates and top with sauce and sautéed vegetables and fruit.

SALMON TANDORI

Makes 4 servings
Juice of one lemon
4 salmon steaks
1 cup of plain, nonfat yogurt
1 (1-inch) piece of fresh ginger, peeled and chopped
2 cloves of garlic, chopped
1 jalapeno pepper, chopped
1 teaspoon of black peppercorns
1 teaspoon of garam masala
1/2 teaspoon of turmeric
Fresh cilantro
4 lemons for garnish

Pour lemon juice over the salmon. Combine the yogurt, ginger, garlic, jalapeno, peppercorns, garam masala, and turmeric in a blender and blend until smooth.

Spoon the mixture over the salmon and refrigerate for at least 4 hours. Preheat the oven to 500 degrees and bake the salmon for 10 minutes, until it flakes easily with a fork.

Garnish it with sprigs of cilantro and serve with lemon wedges.

MEAT

Meats such as beef and lamb provide a great source of protein. Red meat is high in iron and purported to be a sexually potent source of energy. My favorite way to eat meat is Moroccan made in tagine. If you don't want to eat fish, chicken, or vegetarian, then cook your favorite meat dishes; but make sure you use the herbs, spices, and fruits listed under erotic foods to add flavor and pleasure to your meal. However, if you just want a good, plain grilled steak, add some fresh ground pepper, and then pair it with a salad, adding herbs and spices to give it all a great kick.

Here is a sensual recipe that can be used for fish, chicken, meat, or vegetables, the "Spices of Life" to enhance the libido. Prepare the day ahead and put all your love into it.

4 tablespoons of oil
3 whole cloves
Small piece of cinnamon bark
4 green cardamom pods
3 large onions
1 teaspoon of ground cumin
1 teaspoon of coriander
1 teaspoon of ginger
1 teaspoon of turmeric
1 teaspoon of salt

1/2 teaspoon of chili powder
1 pound of meat, fish,
or vegetables 2 teaspoons of fresh mashed garlic
2 teaspoons of basmati rice

Put the oil in a heavy cooking pan and heat. Throw in cloves, cinnamon, and cardamom. After 2 minutes, add chopped onion and cook on medium heat for 5 minutes.

Add all the other spices, except garlic, to the onion mixture.

Cook slowly for 10 minutes, stirring constantly. Add meat, fish, or vegetables and stir to coat with spices. Add garlic. Add enough water to cover ingredients, and for meat or chicken simmer for 1 1/2 hours.

For fish or vegetables, simmer for about 1/2 hour until tender. Cool and refrigerate until the next day.

BREADS

I would purchase a good whole grain bread to go with all the dishes. Use olive oil instead of butter for dipping the bread. The body has a harder time producing testosterone, which is tied to our sex drive, when we cut back on fat. Olive oil is a way to get good fat and a healthy sex drive at the same time. Here is a bread recipe that I found in an old book.

EZEKIEL'S BREAD

This recipe is one of the few specific recipes found in the Bible. Neither Ezekiel nor the people who made and ate the bread realized that they were practicing what is known as "augmentation." It means to pack highly potent grains and quality protein into bread rather than eat bread made of one grain. This bread adds beans to the recipe to give it protein. According to the Bible, the people of the Middle East ate a wide range of beans. Ezekiel's bread is a good source of protein, calcium, phosphorous, iron, potassium, vitamins A and C, thiamin, riboflavin, and niacin.

2 packets of yeast
1/2 cup of warm water
1/3 cup of honey
4 cups of whole wheat flour

2¼ cups of barley flour
1 cup of soy flour
1/4 cup of rye flour
1/2 cup cooked and mashed chickpeas or lentil bears
4 tablespoons of olive oil 2 cups of water
1/2 tablespoon of sea salt

Dissolve yeast in warm water with 1 tablespoon of honey. Set aside for 10 minutes. Combine the next five ingredients. Blend lentils or chickpeas, oil, remaining honey, and a small amount of water in a blender. Place in a large bowl with remaining water. Stir in 1 cup of the mixed flour. Add the yeast mixture. Stir in salt and remaining flour.

Place on floured breadboard and knead until smooth. Put in oiled bowl and let rise until doubled in bulk. Knead again, cut dough, and shape into two loaves. Place in greased pans and let rise. Bake at 375 degrees for 45 minutes to 1 hour.

Note: there is a reference in the passage to adding "fitches," which is a seasoning or herb. It has been suggested that the herbs are cumin, fennel, and nutmeg. If you wish, add 1 teaspoon of cumin, fennel, or nutmeg. These too, along with the chickpeas, make this a sexy bread!

DESSERTS

Of course, anything chocolate, or simply a large chunk of dark rich chocolate to end the meal is sexy. You could pair this with some fresh fruit and a little port. However, I would suggest that you make the following magic cake. You'll recognize that honey, Strega, and the spices are all aphrodisiacs.

HONEY CAKE

Serving honey is an ancient way of honoring guests. Honey was served after the main meal and at the end of the day because it has a calming and tranquilizing effect.

1/2 cup of honey
1/2 cup of Strega wine (or any sweet white wine, but Strega is best)
5 egg yolks
7 egg whites
1½ teaspoons of salt
1 tablespoon of grated orange peel
1/2 cup plus
2 tablespoons olive oil
1 cup whole wheat flour
1/2 teaspoon each of cinnamon, cloves, and nutmeg

Preheat oven to 375 degrees. Whisk egg yolks with honey for five minutes. Add orange peel. Sift flour with salt and spices. Gradually stir in egg yolks and honey. Add wine and olive oil, stirring constantly as you add small amounts. Beat the egg whites until stiff and fold into batter. Line the bottom of an 8-inch spring-form pan with oiled parchment or a brown paper bag cut to size. Oil the pan and paper well. Pour batter into pan and bake for 20 minutes. Turn oven off and let cake sit for 10 minutes. Remove cake from oven. Turn over and detach from spring pan carefully.

Don't forget the wine. A research study from the University of Florence in Italy revealed that those who drank a glass of red wine each day, as opposed to teetotalers, had more natural lubrication and enhanced erections. If you don't want the alcohol, get an alcohol-free grape juice.

THE LOVE FEAST

Now, let's create a love feast. But before we do, let's recap the seven-day plan. First, write down exactly what you want. Be very specific about the love you want in your life. Memorize it and read it aloud every day. Get a rose quartz crystal and do the crystal love spell. Carry the crystal with you. Go into the alpha meditation each morning. Go to my website and you can download free a five-minute meditation video. Listen to the music and allow yourself to relax. Go in the bathroom and do the magic mirror talk. Next, dress with care using jewelry and perfumes to accentuate your sexuality. Do the 15-minute Doctor Lynn's Xercise for a Sexy Body-Mind also found on my website.

Each morning have Cleopatra's drink, and each afternoon have either Casanova's or Don Juan's cocktail. Have a piece of dark rich chocolate every day. Every day have a dropper full of Damiana's Nectar. Choose from the foods, spices, and herbs in the erotic food section of this book for your daily meals. Familiarize yourself with these foods so that when you think about eating you think sexy foods. For example: if you are out at a restaurant and see fava beans on the menu, pick these as well as caviar, fish, and foods with spices and herbs. Shellfish are also a good choice. Use aromatherapy oils and candles to fill your house with sensual scents. Take long, hot bath using aromatherapy oils and candles. Be good to yourself.

On the seventh night, make a love feast. One of the most important things we can do is transform a whole evening into an enchanting love feast. The goal is to create an enchanting atmosphere with ingredients and magical objects that will work their special magic on your guest or on your own ability to draw into your life that which you desire. Here is how I would prepare the love feast. Of course, you should add your own style, so that the romantic evening begins and ends the way you envision it.

Dress the table with pink and green, the colors of Venus, the planet of love. Make a centerpiece of roses, poppies, and bunches of hibiscus, the flowers of love. Make sure you dress in a sexy and alluring manner without being too revealing. Be a bit mysterious. Spray on a nice sexy perfume. Put on soft love music to set the mood.

Basil has long been a traditional herb for love potions and meals. When magically charged, the herb's aura produces a loving sensation within the human body. An hour before your lover comes home, or if by yourself, take two goblets, line them with fresh basil leaves, and then pass a silver coin over the top of each cup, focusing your mind on your lover. Pour a small amount of Strega into the cup and let sit for one hour. When your lover arrives, greet him or her with a small sip of love wine.

Start the meal with either cold strawberry soup in the summer or hot pumpkin soup in the winter. If you don't want soup, serve hummus or another light appetizer. Then make the next course crusty bread with olive oil and a salad of mixed greens and fresh tomatoes and toasted caraway seeds (for lust) with a dressing of balsamic vinegar.

For the main course, how about the apricot chicken or steamed fish with tomatoes, basil, and oregano? Grill or steam fresh asparagus, broccoli, or carrots. Remember the wine, either a good red or white to enhance both the meal and the libido. Beer is also good because it is made from barley, which is ruled by Venus. If you don't want to drink wine have an apple juice cocktail (Don Juan) or drink a hot hibiscus tea.

For dessert, have a slice of magic honey cake, a few slices of fruit, and a piece of dark chocolate. A little glass of port or honey wine with a little cheese and fruit would also be nice.

Remember to charge each piece of the meal with the energy of your love aura before and while you prepare the meal. Don't discount the power of food and ritual to bring love into your life. When lovers meet, one of the first things they do is break bread. They say the way to man's heart is through his stomach. I would say this is true of women as well. Even if your love has not arrived, practice and practice and practice some more, so when he or she does arrive, you will be ready.

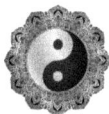

*~ A successful life: to endure hardships
and still be able to laugh. ~*

WHAT IS IT WE ALL DESIRE MOST?

This is such a delicious question and probably stirs up a lot of responses. I decided to explore this question by placing an ad on Craigslist. I explained that I was writing a book. I asked men, first, what it was they desired most. I was surprised at how many men answered the question. I've chosen three answers to share with you.

FIRST RESPONSE:

I think some men want material goods and that is their focus: cars, houses, bank accounts. Some men want a wife and kids and their focus is on providing the comforts of life for them. Although it is possible to have all of the above in some combination, I think the bottom line for me is happiness. My desire is that I'm healthy, and my wife and son are as well. Therefore, to ask what a man desires most is a question with has many answers as there are men.

I think we all desire something a little different depending on where you're at in life. My desires as a young man of 31 are not the same as when I was 21.

I have evolved as a mature gentleman, now my desires are all about family happiness and job satisfaction and the simple pleasures of life. So as a family man I would have to say what I desire most is for my son and daughter to grow into wonderful little/big people that make a positive mark on the world.

Also, that my wife and I remain in love and continue to be happy and healthy together. This is a snapshot of my life at this point.

I hope I was able to provide a small sampling of what this man desires most!

Best, Harlen

SECOND RESPONSE:

At this point in my life, intellect, and what I've termed recently, "curiosity reciprocation," is the most important. In a nutshell, the ability to communicate on topics ranging from debates on String Theory, and theme analysis of Romeo and Juliet to current geopolitical/economic trends would be ideal. However, technical or theoretical intellect is not mandatory, or necessary, for having a loving relationship. What is necessary is that she possesses curiosity and wonder about the world around her.

NATURALLY SEXY & HEALTHY ~ Doctor Lynn Wylnn

* There are changes with age. Generally (as many may suspect),

A.   When younger, physical attributes are the most desirable characteristics, which guide one to pursue a relationship.

B.   When older, genuine companionship, and intellectual stimulation is tantamount (In men who don't mature, the physical may always be the most important).

With men, nationality is not as much of an issue (as I tend to believe it is with women).

I don't think there are dramatic differences with men that are from the U.S., regardless of region. Men outside of the U.S. (particularly Latin and European) possess more promiscuous, predatory sexual natures than men in the U.S. This may hinder and delay the maturity factor, as their tendency to want to conquer supersedes and retards their spiritual maturity growth.

Danny :)

THIRD RESPONSE:

At my age? Peace and good health and a good woman who knows what passion really is. The one you can't keep your hands off or her you. Yes, romance and more!

As a man, I have noticed that I became very sensual so I always seek a woman my age or older as they are the same as me. The young girls do not have the experience or the touch or feel.

Anonymous

I also placed an ad asking for a response from women and no one responded. I trust it might be because of a blind ad Therefore, I will now share a story with you that I think sums it up.

Every woman and every man needs to discover and understand the answer to this riddle if they hope to find and maintain everlasting love.

Love is an emotion with many facets, shades, and colors. The most intense and burning aspect of love is love mixed with deep, passionate, erotic sex. Relationships not blessed with the right mix of love and sex are doomed to fail. Love must be properly balanced with sex, and sex must be properly balanced with love for true happiness to exist. Love alone will not bring happiness to a relationship and nor will just sex. When the two are blended, a relationship has the potential to reach the highest state of passionate lovemaking known to exist on this earthly plane. And when we add the element of romance to the mix, we create an experience that reaches beyond the height of everyday experiences.

It has been said that a woman can make or break a man and a man may easily claim or lose the love of a woman. A true understanding of this statement is the difference between an unhappy chaotic relationship and a relationship that is harmonious. Nagging, bossing, complaining, coldness, and fighting can be traced to a lack of knowledge or ignorance about how to blend the essence of femininity and masculinity when it comes to love, sex, and romance.

Fortunate are the individuals who understand the true relationship between the emotions of love, sex and romance and how they should be played out through the feminine and masculine roles.

The difference between the making and the breaking of a relationship is clear when an understanding of the laws and designs of nature are accepted. The basic "stuff" of the universe is the opposing forces of nature, which can either come together and create or pull apart and destroy. Destruction happens when either force lacks understanding of the nature of its opposing force. When a woman understands and respects masculinity and a man understands and respects femininity, nature allows for the creation of an everlasting union.

If a man or a woman allows their partner to lose interest, or become more interested in other people, it is usually because of ignorance or indifference to understanding the subjects of love, sex, and romance. This, of course, presupposes that true love once existed between the man and the woman.

Partners who argue over trivial matters usually are arguing because of a lack of interest or awareness of the need to fully understand and foster the aspects of love, sex, and romance in a relationship.

Most men, if they would be very honest, would admit that the driving force behind their motivation to excel is that of a woman. The male energy has always been forceful and aggressive, with a need to be the *great hunter*. This is because the great hunter was able to have his pick of any woman in the tribe. He was great because he could provide for her and take care of her needs. This basic instinct has not changed. Rather than animal meat and hides, today's "hunter" seeks money and power as a means of attracting the woman of his desire. Therefore, man's greatest driving force is the desire to please a woman. Without this driving force, power and fortune would be meaningless to most men. It is the desire of a man to please a woman that gives women the power to make or break a man.

The woman who understands the inherent nature of man and, with love and devotion caters to it, will never need to fear other women. Further, although most men would not readily admit to the power held by the woman they desire, the intelligent woman recognizes this aspect of the male ego and wisely makes it a non-issue. She does not wield her power over him. She allows the man his strength and control and seeks to support his need to please rather than try to manipulate him.

The wise man understands that he is greatly influenced by the feminine energy of the woman he desires and intelligently embraces her feminine essence. He understands that without the balancing energy of the right woman he can never be happy and complete. The man who does not understand how to respect and embrace the powerful feminine force of the woman he desires deprives himself of the ability to gain access to a power that has done more to help men achieve greatness than any other force on earth.

Of all the positive emotions we experience, love, sex, romance, and desire head the list. Cynicism must be removed from a person's consciousness in order to make room for these emotions. As long as you live in cynicism, these positive emotions and their experience will elude you. You must not be disappointed if love has not come into your life at this time. It is not easy to believe in finding a true love when you are alone, but if you can let go of the disappointment and stay focused on your desire to find true love, with persistence, love has no choice but to make its way to your heart.

The problem for most people is that they truly don't understand the nature of love. The first step to finding love is to remove all doubt about its existence and believe in it with undying faith even when it does not appear to be anywhere in sight. Those who continue to believe without giving in to settling for the next-best thing (security or to end loneliness) will eventually find the love they seek.

Remember, love is elusive and will not appear until the time is right. If you are alone at this time and searching for your love, remember he or she is not ready to show up now. Be patient and enjoy every element of your life, and when the time is right, you can be sure love will appear. However, you need to be ready and know how to spot it when it arrives. In this book, hopefully you discovered the fundamental steps that will put you into the right place at the right time to meet your true love.

The 7th-century text for *Tantra* and an ancient Arthurian legend give us an answer to this riddle of just what it is we all desire most.

To understand fully this ancient riddle about desire and love, you must fully understand the underlying meaning.

Ancient texts, like most of life's questions and answers, are allegorical in nature, meaning that behind most every question and answer in life is often a hidden meaning that once revealed will give insight into the essential nature of things.

A riddle is described as a puzzling question requiring some ingenuity to answer. Who would depute that the relationship between a man and a woman is not, at times, a puzzling question requiring great ingenuity? If men and women could really understand the essence of each other, there would be far less room for conflict. With egos aside and openness to understanding, the essential elements that create a harmonious relationship are what will bring about a deep and lasting love into your life.

Love requires that we be clever and resourceful. It is not enough to simply find the answers to life's most puzzling question (love). You must be willing to understand fully the meaning and then be able to apply the principles to your life. Relationships are contrasting. Masculinity always contrasts with femininity, as femininity always contrasts with masculinity. The only way to understand the nature of relationships is to fully understand and appreciate the contrasting nature. Insight into the yin and the yang of attraction and love brings this appreciation.

The ancient riddle to finding love and beauty is simple. It lies at the heart of discovering the female essence and the masculinity of manhood. It is not about power or control, but about discovering how the right to make decisions and act according to the inherent essence of your sexual being brings the most passionate and liberating expression of true love.

The riddle is simple but the answer takes some thought.

What is it a woman and a man desire most?

This riddle may best be answered by looking at the female essence. In the 7th century AD in India, mystical texts called *Tantras* began to personify women as divinity and as the vital breath of the universe. For almost the first time since the establishment of the Indo-European male-centered systems of worship, females were worshiped as being supreme. Shakti, personified by Kali, the female goddess, is seen whirling around her husband in a dance of destruction as she rides his body in sexual ecstasy. It indicates her enjoyment of erotic games and her determination to exert her own will in the area of sexuality.

Although Kali or Shiva is sometimes mistakenly portrayed as bloodthirsty in character and appearance, her actions were never meant to be destructive. On the contrary, she was meant to be portrayed as wiping out the demonic forces before they could destroy the universe. She was symbolic of empowerment for women. She portrayed the perfect model of power and balance and was actively assertive rather than pointlessly destructive. She returned to women the three virtues that had been historically denied them: strength (moral and physical), intellect (knowledge and wisdom) and sexual sovereignty.

Assertiveness is one of the most obvious qualities given to women deities who embody the female essence. It was likewise the main theme of the Arthurian legend of Gawain and Ragnell. Sir Gawain was one of the most handsome and popular knights of the age. He agreed to marry a loathsome hag named Ragnell in return for the answer to this riddle; what does a woman desire most?

Most of the retelling of this story has made it seem that what a woman wants most is to have her own way always and forever. However, the truth of the story is different. When, on the night of their marriage, Gawain kissed the hideous and ugly hag Ragnell out of sense of pity, she immediately turned into a beautiful woman. Secretly, she had wanted Gawain to kiss her in her ugliness, because if he did, the curse that was bestowed upon her would be removed and she would become a beautiful woman. But because he kissed her out of a sense of pity and not from desire, the curse was only partly removed.

Ragnell then offered Gawain a choice: she would stay beautiful either by day when they would appear in public or by night when they were alone. Gawain told Ragnell he could not decide and that he would leave the decision up to her. In this way, he gave her sovereignty over herself. Sovereignty is the answer to the riddle. Gawain passed the test of manhood and chivalry, and Ragnell rewarded him by remaining beautiful forever.

Therefore, it seems that what both a man and a woman desire the most is sovereignty—the power to choose. *Sovereignty* is the quality or authority of being independent and in charge of the conditions you live under.

Sovereignty carries with it **responsibility**. That is, if you take your life in your own hands, you also take it upon yourself to act responsibly and with integrity in regards to your own life, your family, your community, your fellow human beings and the planet as a whole. You respect the very nature and differences between man and woman with an intellectual understanding of what it takes to find and maintain true love.

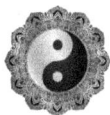

*~ A successful life: finally giving yourself
the freedom to really live. ~*

CONCLUSION

The conclusion for most authors, I believe, is bittersweet. This is the end of a long journey. There is tremendous satisfaction, and at the same time, there is a sadness that the end of such a passionate venture is in sight. However, like love, lust, and sex, the ending of one phase opens the door to another phase.

Awareness is the ultimate key to happiness and to fulfilling sex. Awareness bridges the gap between momentary pleasure and a deeper understanding of the nature of sacred sexuality. You may read a list of things to do to improve your sex life, but when you add the element of understanding, you relate in a way that gets to the heart of passion. Reading this book you are now aware of the foods, herbs, spices, exercises, scents, colors, words, flirts, and gestures that will bring to you the love and the sexual energy you desire. However, knowledge is not enough. You must understand what it all means. Awareness gives you the ability to absorb life to the fullest. With knowledge and understanding, even the most trivial everyday occurrences make life more meaningful and connect us with the "here and now."

Every thought, every action, and every word you convey has a direct effect on your lovemaking. The purpose of this book was to open up your awareness to the natural things around you that not only enhance your sexual self but also enhance your life. When we add emotion to insight and knowledge, we experience passion. Self-confidence replaces negative patterns and resistance to change. With awareness, people discover their own power, making the sexual experience spontaneous and exhilarating.

Vigorous sex requires a healthy body-mind. Physical fitness and stamina are best achieved through diet and exercise. Specific foods and specific exercises work wonders for your sex life. The sex drive for almost everyone is a switch that can be changed from negative to positive. It just takes awareness and implementation of healthy habits along with a healthy attitude.

We all have experienced that rush of sexual excitement that comes about when we meet someone new. The passion, the physical affection, and the stolen moments when you are sure this will last forever. Sadly, life can get in the way. Marriage or a long-term relationship often gives way to complacency, boredom, and reality. Work, children, responsibility, and familiarity all play havoc on our sexual passion. Add sickness, exhaustion, and the pressures and stresses of modern-day life, and is it any wonder sex fades?

Therefore, we search endlessly for aphrodisiacs and answers that, quite honestly, are right under our noses. Common sense is a powerful tool when it come to love, sex, and simply living a healthy and satisfying life. Sex is such a major part of our lives. Sex sells, sex gets our attention, sex makes us feel good, and sex is the driving force behind success.

Our spirit and our sexuality are forces that are present within us from birth to death. With creativity, we can create a limitless relationship that unfolds and expands beyond the everyday experience. With awareness, lovers can intensify the experiences of sex through sight, sound, taste, smell, touch, and intuition. With this kind of intimate exploration, sex is never boring, and infidelity is inconceivable. With respect and insight, each person becomes, over and over again, a new person, keeping the relationship fresh and alive. It begins with you. It begins with good habits that include diet, exercise, and the removal of addictive and negative behaviors.

True lovers become experts at turning each other on. They encourage, support, understand, and give as much as they take. Love is the essential ingredient that makes sex more than simply a physical release. Love is binding. It carries us from one stage in life to another and from one generation to another.

There are no guarantees when it comes to love. Love may come more than once in your lifetime, but there will be one love that will stand above the rest. If you find this love, cherish it, feed it, and keep it. Don't be cynical if it should part. Giving someone all your love is never an assurance that he or she will love you back. So, when you love, don't expect love in return. Love is whimsical. It comes and goes as it pleases. Every person who has been moved by love knows that whether it stays or goes, it imprints an indelible mark on the soul. It endures long after the object of one's desire has faded away.

Now, if you feel yourself unfortunate to have loved and lost, perish the thought. If you have loved truly, you have never lost. Be content that you experienced love in your heart. When I was young, I fell madly in love. I truly loved this man with all my heart. I thought he loved me, too; but alas, he did not — not in the way I loved him. It hurt me dearly, and I spent many years in sadness until, one day, I realized that I had felt love. I had experienced what it was like to be deeply in love. Many people never take this chance. I was lucky to have the experience. I knew what love felt like. And even though it did not last, I would not have wanted to live my life without those feelings and that experience.

Love comes more than once into your life. Love may come and go a number of times. Don't be disappointed if it should depart. No force that touches the human heart with such passion as love can possibly be harmful except through ignorance.

Love is an emotion with many shades, sides, colors, and configurations. But the most intense form of love is that which is blended with sex and romance. When these three things are blended, we experience what is known as spiritual love. This is love and sex at its best. In this book, I've presented you with ways to bring love, sex, and romance into your life. It begins with you.

The definition of an aphrodisiac is an agent (food or drug) that arouses or is held to arouse sexual desires. It is something that excites. Humans have always searched for the magic elixir of life that would bring eternal happiness, love, sex, health, power, and wealth. Self-confidence, a healthy lifestyle, passion, caring, understanding, playfulness, and respect are mighty aphrodisiacs when it comes to excitement and arousal.

Sometimes, exactly what we desire is right in front of us. Awareness is the key. If sex is as much about health as it is about being aroused, then live healthfully and be well. If great sex is about understanding and knowing, then maturity and experience should bring you the wisdom to understand the difference between love and lust. Lust never lasts but true love endures.

Don't look for things to be easy. A relationship is work just like all things in life. However, it can be a labor of love, with the right attitude. Your attitude is the way you look at something. With a positive attitude toward love, relationships, and sex, the experience reaches beyond the ordinary and into the extraordinary. It is in our nature to constantly want more and better, and yet more and better are simply constructs that can be found in the simplest of things. A kiss can be more and can be better with the right attitude. A touch can be fulfilling and sex can be more satisfying when we apply an attitude of giving more, rather than seeking more. It is so easy to stop trying and move on to the next conquest, but one thing I have learned is that all relationships take work.

Sex always dwindles with familiarity and time. It ebbs and flows. The intelligent person understands this and works hard to keep the sexual fires burning. It does not take a lot of money, vacations, or new partners. What it does take is love, caring, and the ability to reach out with compassion. It takes a deep understanding of the true essence of love and how love can always bring us back to a place of lovemaking as opposed to just sex.

The search for aphrodisiacs and love potions that will make another person love us against their own will is always the wrong approach to finding everlasting love. Love is something that grows, and with this growth, comes the potential to experience sex beyond what words can describe.

Bhakti yoga describes a relationship as being that which dances on the "razor's edge." It means that if we slip and fall into either a position of too much closeness or too much separateness we damage (cut) ourselves and the relationship. There must be balance. In order to maintain our balance we need to come back to the moment constantly. This involves a jolt from our fantasies and daydreams and a stepping into the present moment. In the present moment, we have the opportunity to start fresh — to see our lover or the potential to find our lover as new and exciting. Retreating into fantasy, we get stuck in hopes and images with unreal expectations.

Dancing on the razor's edge means including and embracing all of a relationship. Even in anger, if we can embrace love, the pain and the loneliness of the moment subside. In the uncertainty of the moment, whether you are in a relationship or not, it is the realization that we do not need to be stuck by settling into one way or another. Each moment has the opportunity to bring a renewed sense of energy and a renewed sense of love.

Being prepared for love with an open mind assures that it will find its way into your life. Sadly, the truth is that we are all quite self-centered and we spend a great deal of time trying to control one another and life so that we can get what we want. If we can admit this to ourselves, we can set about the alchemical work of transforming the lead of the ego and attachments into the gold of surrender and love.

Sexuality should be sacred. It is the art and discipline of turning sex into lovemaking where we experience the unconditional love as the ultimate reality. It is based upon the view that the sexual energy is sacred and precious and not to be squandered away.

Orgasm is the closest simulation to the experience of bliss, which the ancient scriptures of Hinduism tell us we are all ultimately striving to experience. However, the orgasmic experience is only a drop of energy in the experience of bliss, and of course, it is fleeting. The momentary experience of an orgasm creates a moment of balance, but the balance does not last. Love extends this balance.

Our attitude toward sacred sexuality is something that must be cultivated even when we are not engaging in sexual activity. The ultimate experience is when we treat each other with respect, not just when we want something, but simply as a byproduct of unconditional love. The success of our sexual union depends upon our attitude toward life as a whole.

Through all I have experienced in my life, I have learned that the greatest aphrodisiac of all is the one that begins with you. It is your attitude, your energy, self-love, pride in appearance, confidence, awareness, and understanding laced with compassion for all of life. A sexually charged person walks with a confident and self-assured gait. A sexually charged person has a warm smile, a gentle touch, and an energy that light up a room. It all begins with awareness and then taking the steps to apply what you know to what you want to achieve. I hope that this book has opened your mind to what it means to find the alchemists' Philosopher's Stone — the essence of life — the essence of sexuality.

In closing, let me share with you some of the things I have learned over the years.

Sex doesn't die out in every marriage or relationship. Sex has its ups and its downs. It can always be refreshed and invigorated. It is more than the act. A friend of mine told me a story about his father and mother who had a very passionate relationship. He happened to witness a touching scene. His father was dying and his mother stood by his bed. He reached his hand out and laid it on her breast. They kissed and embraced. They made love.

In every relationship, you will argue and, sometimes, fight. It's all in how you argue and how you fight that determine the outcome, which ultimately should be make-up sex. There will be times when you can't stand each other and you need space. It's okay to take some space, to pull back and breathe. It won't last if you truly love each other.

Don't share everything. It's okay to have little secrets as long as they are not detrimental to the relationship. It's okay to have privacy. It's okay to be you as a separate entity. In fact, it's healthy.

Always try to look nice. Treat your partner as if they are someone special. Dress to excite and please. Even when I was in bed and in pain healing from my cancer surgery I put on a pretty robe, combed my hair, and put on a little makeup. Grooming shows you care. Remember, we are all visual creatures.

Tell the truth. Be honest with each other. Withholding the truth, even if it is a struggle to express, will only hurt you

NATURALLY SEXY & HEALTHY ~ Doctor Lynn Wylnn

both in the end. However, remember to do no harm. Tell the truth from a place of compassion and understanding.

Don't try to change the other person. Learn to accept and not get caught up in the minutia. When you accept a person for who they are and learn to let things go, you will find humor rather than irritation. A friend of mine who is in his late 80s and has been married to the same woman since he was in his 30s told me that the secret to a happy marriage is to ignore 80% of what happens, but make sure you understand the 20% that is important and you pay close attention to it.

Respect, appreciate, and acknowledge each other. These three things will get you through anything. Without respect, appreciation, and acknowledgment, it is impossible to maintain a loving relationship. If these three things are missing, get out! It's not worth the aggravation!

Get outside help when needed but don't rely too heavily on counseling. Many marriages have ended after counseling. Make sure you are going to get help for the right reasons. If the counselor does not understand and is not taking you in the right direction, leave the councilor and find someone new.

Leave if you're not happy and cannot make the person you are with happy. Staying together for children or money is never an answer. If you must cheat, lie, and disrespect, then for everyone's sake, it is time to move on.

Love does come more than once in your life. Don't be cynical because you loved and lost. Take care of yourself, as I have suggested in this book, and love will find its way to your door.

Go out on dates. Make special time to have fun. It does not take a lot of money to plan time together — a dinner at home, a movie, or a walk in nature holding hands. Make time to make the relationship special.

Share the burden. Make sure you both share the responsibility of the relationship and the work. If one must carry more than the other carries, be kind, considerate, and do what you can to make things easier.

Never say anything or do anything flirtatious with another man or woman that you wouldn't do in front of your partner. It reminds you that you have integrity.

Make sure you have shared values and compatibilities. Sex has its ups and downs, but compatibility and shared values are the foundation that keeps a relationship intact. Carefully examine the level of your compatibilities. Trust me; these can take relationships from hot to cold. It's important to look at lifestyle choices. Marrying for money, loneliness, wanting security, family pressures, or for whatever reason other than compatibility and shared values, is a mistake. It will only bring you unhappiness and loneliness.

With all the other things in place, make sure you are incredibly sexually attracted to your partner. None of this "this is a nice person; this person will make a good husband, wife, mother, father, they have money, or status" will matter much if the spark of chemistry is missing. If you have that kind of spark that lights up when the other person enters a room, even years after you've been together, consider yourself lucky. It's not easy to find, but it is the basis that will keep you connected through all the perils of life.

And remember this: never, ever lose your sense of humor! Because in the end there is only one thing that counts — "Was it fun?"

I spent 25 years searching for my soul mate. In those 25 years, I had many relationships. Some good and some, well, not so good. Each time I walked away knowing deep in my heart it was not the right relationship and not wanting to hurt another person, I did not give in to the loneliness. I employed all the methods given in this book, and although it took years to find my soul mate, it did happen. I watched many of my friends over the years marry and divorce or end up in unhappy relationships. My marriage is not perfect, and we have had our share of problems. We've worked hard, but at the heart of it all we have that intense chemistry mixed with compatibility, respect, caring, and compassion.

Love, sexuality, and romance mixed together bring a passion for life.

When it is all said and done, there are only two things that you take with you: the love you have given and the love you have received.

Sex does matter and pleasure is so delightful...it's a natural thing.

Doctor Lynn

A SUCCESSFUL LIFE IS...

Having no regrets about the things you wish you had done, instead to focus on all the things you have done.

And I would add a few more to the successful life list: a lifelong best friend, being a grandparent, to have touched with love another human being in body, mind and soul, laugh often and hear those you love laugh often and the most important thing of all...have fun because, in the end, there is only one question to ask:

Was it fun?

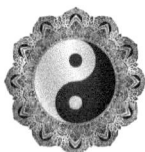

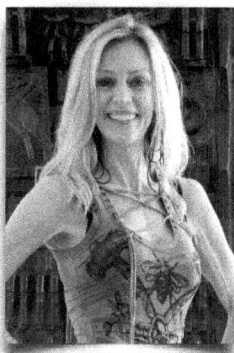

ABOUT THE AUTHOR

Born on a small island off the coast of Maine, Doctor Lynn grew up in a small village where folk medicine was routinely practiced. She left the island as a young single mother on welfare to enter college at the University of Maine. She graduated with a degree in Communication and then went on to study Naturopathy, Aromatherapy, Herbology, Yoga therapy and Fitness affiliation with ACE. She has over 30 years' of experience in teaching, writing and producing books and videos on how to stay healthy, happy, find wealth and discover Inner wisdom of your body, mind and soul. Her inspiring life journey from her humble beginnings to a wealthy world traveler, published author, international speaker, TV and DVD producer, Doctor Lynn will share with you what it takes to live a healthy, wealthy, happy and peaceful life in your body, mind and soul.

Doctor Lynn lives in Sarasota, Florida with her husband Dan. She is the mother of two children; Derek and Kristen, and the grandmother of three; Gareth, Sam and Mia who give her the greatest joy in life.

Visit the author online at:
DoctorLynn.com